Oligonucleotides - Overview and Applications

Edited by Arghya Sett

Published in London, United Kingdom

Oligonucleotides - Overview and Applications
http://dx.doi.org/10.5772/intechopen.104311
Edited by Arghya Sett

Contributors
Michael Hausmann, Eberhard Schmitt, Melissa J. LaBonte, Jamie Z. Roberts, Mikio Nishizawa, Tetsuya Okuyama, Richi Nakatake, Elena Kalinichenko, Kristen L. Rhinehardt, Eugene Uwiragiye, Arghya Sett

First published in London, United Kingdom, 2023 by IntechOpen
IntechOpen is the global imprint of INTECHOPEN LIMITED, registered in England and Wales, registration number: 11086078, 5 Princes Gate Court, London, SW7 2QJ, United Kingdom

British Library Cataloguing-in-Publication Data
A catalogue record for this book is available from the British Library

Additional hard and PDF copies can be obtained from orders@intechopen.com

Oligonucleotides - Overview and Applications
Edited by Arghya Sett
p. cm.
Print ISBN 978-1-80355-627-7
Online ISBN 978-1-80355-628-4
eBook (PDF) ISBN 978-1-80355-629-1

Meet the editor

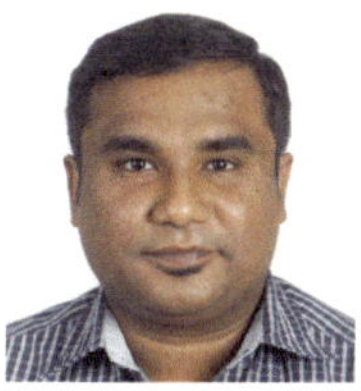

Arghya Sett is a researcher in biotechnology who strives for the integration of technology in biomedical research. He is currently a postdoc research scientist at the Institute of Organic Chemistry and Biochemistry (IOCB), Prague, and the Czech Academy of Sciences (AS CR). He obtained a Ph.D. from the Indian Institute of Technology Guwahati (IIT Guwahati), India. His research involved how the aptamer-a molecule can help in molecular diagnostics for breast cancer. After obtaining his degree, Dr. Sett continued his research at the University of Bordeaux, France, where he developed light-up aptamers to detect pre-micro RNAs for muscular dystrophy and aptasensors to detect small molecules. He is a dynamic researcher and active in collaborative research. He has published more than eleven research articles, several review articles, and three book chapters. He has also filed three patents in India. He actively participates and presents his research work at international conferences and symposiums. His research on the development of low-cost diagnostics has attracted media attention and garnered him several accolades.

Contents

Preface

Oligonucleotides are comprised of nucleoside bases, sugars, and triphosphates. These nucleic acids are biological macromolecules found in all life forms encoding genetic information.

The chemical composition of nucleic acids was extensively studied in the early 1900s and five nucleotide bases including uracil have been identified. Although the elemental compositions were known, the correct structures were not established until the chemical synthesis of nucleotides was performed. Following various milestone inventions by eminent scientists like Emil Fischer and Albert Kossel, James Watson, Francis Crick, and Rosalind Franklin discovered the double helical structure of DNA, for which Watson and Crick were awarded the Nobel Prize. This discovery helped to solve the most significant biological riddle of the time and advance oligonucleotide-based research.

In recent decades, a plethora of modified nucleotides have been synthesized using nucleic acid chemistry. These molecules have proved to be useful for gene therapy and DNA-based diagnostics. Diverse forms of structures, chemistries, and mechanisms of action exist for oligonucleotide-based therapeutics. These drug candidates target either mRNAs or proteins. Antisense oligonucleotides (ASOs), siRNAs, antagomirs, splice-switching oligonucleotides, and DNAzymes target mainly RNA moiety, while immunostimulatory sequences and aptamers target proteins. The recent approval of many oligonucleotide-based drug candidates is indicative of the extensive vitality of the field. The unique base-pairing properties of nucleic acids have already been exploited to develop biosensors for disease diagnosis. The ability of single-stranded oligonucleotides or aptamers to self-assemble into complex structures may possess enormous potential in future nanoscale engineering and DNA-based computing. This book discusses the various biological processes targeted and the corresponding oligonucleotide interventions. It includes six chapters that discuss new developments in modified oligonucleotides and various theranostic applications of oligonucleotides.

I would like to give my heartfelt thanks to all the authors and contributors as well as the staff at IntechOpen. I believe that the case studies of modified bases, cutting-edge fluorescence in situ hybridization (FISH) technology and other techniques discussed in this book will provide guidance and support to researchers in the field as well as future developers in the oligonucleotide industry.

Arghya Sett
Postdoc Research Scientist,
Institute of Organic Chemistry and Biochemistry,
Czech Academy of Sciences,
Prague, Czech Republic

Section 1

Introduction

Chapter 1

Introductory Chapter: Oligonucleotides – Overview and Applications

Arghya Sett

1. Introduction

Oligonucleotides are polymers of nucleic acids which are building blocks of life. It is one of the key elements of the central dogma of life. Any nucleotide consists of a pentose sugar (ribose in case of RNA and de-oxy ribose for DNA), a phosphate group and any one nitrogenous base (nine-member double ring bases adenine, guanine as purines and six-membered single ring base thymine, uracil and cytosine as pyrimidines). On basis of structure and stability, researchers are working to expand the genetic alphabets [1]. This will extend the diversity of the oligonucleotides and demystification of mystical doctrine like "RNA world hypothesis" [2].

2. Applications

2.1 Oligo-based therapeutics

Oligonucleotides have several applications from encoding, transmitting and expressing genetic information to storage of information, disease diagnostics and even oligonucleotide-based therapeutics. As DNA, RNA is omnipresent in our body, due to its non-immunogenicity, and it also easily be exploited as cargo for drug delivery at specific locations of cellular organelles.

Among whole proteome of our body, only 10–14% of proteins have active binding sites which are "druggable" [3]. To address this issue, nucleic acid-based strategies can exploit translational machinery of the mammalian cells. Antisense oligonucleotides (ASOs) like short single-stranded DNA, phosphorothioate DNA, siRNAs, micro RNAs and locked nucleic acids are key players in drug development processes. There is plethora of ASO-based drugs approved by FDA against several diseases like Duchenne Muscular Dystrophy (DMD), viral diseases, Type2 diabetes, cancer and others. However, poor cellular uptake and rapid degradation or renal filtration DNA-based therapeutics needs modification of delivery module to facilitate internalization and retain their active form [4].

2.2 Oligo-based sensing methods

Besides the carrier of genetic information, breakthroughs in DNA-based biotechniques, CRISPR-based gene editing and other tools revolutionized the nucleotide-based sensing platforms. Among these sensing techniques, PCR, RT-PCR, antisense technology, single nucleotide polymorphisms in cancer and other deadly genetic disorders played an important role and often been converted into convenient biosensors. In the current COVID pandemic era, DNA-based POC diagnostics played a critical role in early and rapid detection of viral infections and followed to better patient management [5]. Even, to combat the urgent medical emergencies against SARS-CoV2, synthetic DNA-based vaccine was a lifesaver in the process of vaccine development. These nucleotide-based vaccines are amenable to scale-up, cheaper, cold-chain free stable, which are of critical attributes for delivery to resource-limited spaces.

Oligonucleotides having specific target binding or catalytic functions are termed as "Functional DNA". Such an example of functional DNA is "Aptamers", also called "Magic bullets" are considered to be chemical equivalent of monoclonal antibodies for their specificity and sensitivity to their cognate targets [6]. The target repertoire is diverse ranging from small molecules, metabolites, to proteins, cell surface receptors, cells and tissues and even whole organisms. Another major variant of functional DNA is ribozymes or deoxy ribozymes which are analogues of enzymes having specific recognition sites and cleavage activity. They also catalyze certain biochemical reactions. Due to stability, specificity, and variability for the base-pairing hybridization for detection and diagnosis, oligonucleotide-based biosensors are the key shareholder in clinical diagnosis, genome mutation detection and environmental pollutant detection [7, 8].

Recent developments in DNA nanotechnology include advent of various modified functional DNAs (XNAs), DNA computing, logic gates, DNA-based signal amplification strategy which further extended the applications of DNA-based sensors in POC detection, live cell imaging and monitoring, disease prognosis and overall, in health management systems [9].

This book presents a collection of new developments in modified oligonucleotides, cutting edge theranostic applications of oligonucleotides which provide insights and comprehensive overview of this exciting topic to the scientific community.

Author details

Arghya Sett
Institute of Organic Chemistry and Biochemistry, Czech Academy of Sciences, Prague, Czech Republic

*Address all correspondence to: arghya.sett@gmail.com

References

[1] Kimoto M, Hirao I. Genetic alphabet expansion technology by creating unnatural base pairs. Chemical Society Reviews. 2020;**49**(21):7602-7626

[2] Neveu M, Kim HJ, Benner SA. The "strong" RNA world hypothesis: Fifty years old. Astrobiology. 2013;**13**(4):391-403

[3] Halgren TA. Identifying and characterizing binding sites and assessing druggability. Journal of chemical information and modeling. 2009;**49**(2):377-389

[4] Dhuri K, Bechtold C, Quijano E, Pham HT, Gupta A, Vikram A, et al. Antisense oligonucleotides: An emerging area in drug discovery and development. Journal of Clinical Medicine. 2020;**9**:2004

[5] Gary EN, Weiner DB. DNA vaccines: Prime time is now. Current Opinion in Immunology. 2020;**65**:21-27

[6] Sett A. Aptamers: Magic bullet for Theranostic applications. In: Theranostics-an Old Concept in New Clothing. London, UK: IntechOpen; 2020

[7] Dong Y, Yao C, Zhu Y, Yang L, Luo D, Yang D. DNA functional materials assembled from branched DNA: Design, synthesis, and applications. Chemical Reviews. 2020;**120**(17):9420-9481

[8] Sett A, Das S, Bora U. Functional nucleic-acid-based sensors for environmental monitoring. Applied Biochemistry and Biotechnology. 2014;**174**:1073-1091

[9] Seeman NC, Sleiman HF. DNA nanotechnology. Nature Reviews Materials. 2017;**3**(1):1-23

Section 2

Modified Oligonucleotides

Chapter 2

The Importance of the Fifth Nucleotide in DNA: Uracil

Jamie Z. Roberts and Melissa J. LaBonte

Abstract

Uracil is a ribonucleotide found in both DNA and RNA, with the main difference between the two being the presence of thymine in DNA and uracil in RNA. Although thymine and uracil are similar in function and can form the same base pairs with adenine, the presence of uracil in DNA can affect DNA stability and modulate cell-specific functions. Without repair mechanisms to remove uracil from DNA, cytosine deamination can occur, resulting in gene drift that is not tolerable in organisms. While the deamination of cytosine in DNA signals damage, a corresponding deamination in RNA would yield normal RNA constituents. To correct this, uracil DNA glycosylases detect and remove uracil bases from uracil-containing DNA, but not natural thymine-containing DNA. The mechanisms of uracil incorporation into DNA, its roles in DNA, cellular mechanisms to detect and remove uracil, and the clinical utility of uracil in DNA will be discussed in this chapter.

Keywords: uracil, uracil-DNA glycosylase, cytosine deaminase, DNA integrity, DNA damage, base excision repair

1. Introduction

Conservation of DNA integrity is important during replication to ensure that daughter cells have accurately replicated DNA to promote genetic continuity. The accumulation of aberrations within the DNA sequence, if left unrepaired, can lead to genetic drift and subsequent detrimental effects following subsequent rounds of replication. Given that the rate of DNA replication occurs at a frequency of 500 nucleotides/minute/replication fork, only a small number of errors (~1 nucleotide per 1×10^9 nucleotides) arise during the replication process [1]. Evolution has enabled the cell to develop proof-reading mechanisms that minimise the potential disruption and preservation of its genetic code [2, 3]; however, errors remain and with time contribute to increased genomic instability and an altered metabolic landscape as required for a sufficient supply of macromolecules, including nucleotides, to drive proliferation [4–6].

Uracil is one of the most frequently occurring error bases in DNA, occurring through mutagen hydrolytic deamination of cytosine to uracil or through substantial uracil DNA misincorporation, and the cell has, therefore, evolved different strategies to target and repair this type of DNA damage. In the absence of uracil-DNA repair, relatively fast cytosine deamination and the toxicity of the resulting uracil will result in a gene drift which is likely not tolerated by an organism.

2. Evolution of the genome: why thymine was key

The genome of all organisms on earth today is coded by 4 nucleobases, which are the two purines, adenine (A) and guanine (G), and the 2 pyrimidines, cytosine (C) and thymine (T). The nucleobases are commonly conjugated to (deoxy)ribose, which are termed nucleosides, and they can then be further conjugated to phosphate groups, giving them the name nucleotides. As deoxynucleotide triphosphates (dNTPs), the nucleobases A, T, G and C are commonly incorporated into DNA, held in a sequence via covalent attachments to the DNA backbone (made up of covalently attached deoxyribose and phosphate in a chain), making a DNA strand. A DNA strand is paired with another DNA strand (forming the classic double-helix structure of DNA) which are complementary to one another via hydrogen bonds between nucleobases within adjacent strands of the DNA helix. In 'normal' DNA, A:T and G:C always pair with one another. Uracil (U) is another nucleobase that is mostly found in RNA, which is synthesised via nucleotide triphosphates (NTPs). RNA can form similar structures to DNA, except that A:U pair together instead of A:T and that the RNA backbone incorporates ribose instead of deoxyribose. RNA is also able to encode genetic information (mRNA) but is more diverse and carries out functions similar to proteins (tRNA and ribozymes). One might ask what the need is for these two similar systems for carrying genetic information and why are they different? To answer these questions, it helps to explore the evolution of the genome.

Life on earth is thought to have originated ~3.8 billion years ago from what is termed the 'primordial soup' (or prebiotic soup). In this prebiotic world the 'RNA world' hypothesis states that the first complex organic molecules to form were RNA based. To support this hypothesis, analysis of carbonaceous meteorites that have fallen to earth have found to contain a range of carbon-molecules, including U, A and G (but not C), which is thought to represent the composition of a very young earth (reviewed here [7]). Additionally, a formamide-based scenario has purposed that formamide (available in the prebiotic earth [8]) could be the starting point for generating all the RNA-components, under conditions that are thought to be present in the prebiotic earth, with U being generated in good yield [9–12]. This leads to the belief that the hereditary genetic information might have been RNA. It is thought that, eventually, there was transition to a DNA-based hereditary system since the deoxyribose-containing DNA backbone is much more stable than ribose-containing RNA backbone [13–15] and RNA replication seems to be far more error prone than DNA replication [16]. In turn, this allowed the evolution of larger, more complex genomes and, therefore, complex multicellular organisms to form.

Potentially, at some point RNA and other molecules were concentrated in a membrane-like structure (making certain catalytic reactions feasible), forming the first RNA cells with metabolism. RNA can catalyse reactions (ribozymes), encode genetic information, transport amino acids (tRNA) and catalyse peptide-bond formation (ribosomes). The idea that RNA was first to carry out these critical functions of the cell is based on ribosomal RNA being extensively involved in peptide-bond formation, suggesting that proteins potentially became essential later in evolution [17]. To allow for the transition from an RNA to DNA cell, the evolution of a mechanism to convert NTPs (containing ribose) to dNTPs (containing deoxyribose) must have occurred. Ribonucleotide reductases (RNRs) frequently catalyses the conversion of nucleotide diphosphates (NDP)/NTP in eukaryotic/prokaryotic cells into dNDP/dNTP, respectively, and are thought to have a common ancestor [18, 19]. Interestingly, it is thought that the first DNA cell would have incorporated U (instead of T) into its genome. This is backed up by the fact that RNR can directly convert ATP, UTP, GTP and CTP into its corresponding dNTPs; however, dTTP needs extra steps involving deoxyuridine monophosphate (dUMP) conversion to dTMP, via thymidylate synthase (TS or TYMS), and two phosphorylation steps by kinases to produce dTTP [20]. Due to this convoluted route to produce dTTP, yet dUTP is synthesised in a simpler manner, it would make sense in an evolutionary context that the initial DNA cell first incorporated U into its DNA, which was then later replaced by T.

One might ask why the need of T-based DNA when U-based DNA performs the same task and is energetically easier to make? C deamination produces U, which happens at a relatively fast rate. A deaminated C will produced a G:U mismatch and led to mutated DNA during replication. In U-based DNA, a U produced via C deamination and U that is normally incorporated in DNA are chemically identical and, therefore, a G:U mismatch would be difficult to identify as damaged DNA, in the context of primitive cells without sophisticated DNA repair mechanisms. To overcome this issue, cells evolved to incorporate T instead of U into their DNA, making U produced from C deamination completely foreign instead. This meant that T-based DNA produced more stable genomes, which is especially important for evolving and maintaining large complex genomes found in, for example, multicellular organisms.

For T-based DNA to be viable, the cell evolved three key enzymes: dUTP nucleotidohydrolase (dUTPase), thymidylate synthase (TS) and uracil-DNA glycosylases (UDGs). After dUTP synthesis via RNR, dUTP is potently dephosphorylated to dUMP by dUTPase. In a two-fold mechanism, this reduces dUTP levels, reducing U misincorporation into the DNA, and produces the TS substrate (dUMP, as discussed in the previous paragraph), leading to an increase in dTTP. The relative levels of the dUTP:dTTP pools determines the rate of U misincorporation into DNA, due to DNA polymerase having difficulty distinguishing between dTTP and dUTP, which are identical molecules except for a single methyl group. In fact, DNA polymerases readily incorporate dUTP as well as dTTP based on their representative concentration and nucleotide availability [21]. If U is misincorporated or C deamination occurs, a UDG removes U, creating an abasic site where no nucleobase is present in a strand of DNA, and a primitive form of DNA damage repair could have corrected it. With the evolution of these 3 proteins, cells were able to detect C deamination (which is always mutagenic) rapidly, repair it and reduce U misincorporation as well.

3. Biosynthesis of NTPs

Nucleotide synthesis *begins with U*(ridine monophosphate) and *I*(nosine monophosphate) [22–24]. The success of DNA replication is dependent upon a number of factors including the availability of balanced nucleotide pools and the cellular ability to recognise misincorporated bases in DNA and initiate their removal and subsequent repair. In the quiescent state, the genomic content of the cell is at its' minimum. Following stimulation to enter the cell cycle and initiate S-phase, DNA biosynthesis is up-regulated and therefore access to the required deoxynucleotide triphosphates (dNTPs) is vital for errorless replication of the genetic material [25]. The enzyme ribonucleotide reductase (RNR) is the initiating factor that induces the reduction of ribonucleoside diphosphates into their respective deoxyribonucleoside diphosphates (dNDPs) [26, 27]. Additional phosphorylation of the nucleosides occurs through the action of nucleoside diphosphate kinase (NDPK), converting the dNDP's to dNTP. However, the synthesis of dTTP requires additional steps within the biosynthesis pathway (**Figure 1**; for an in-depth review, see ref. [28]).

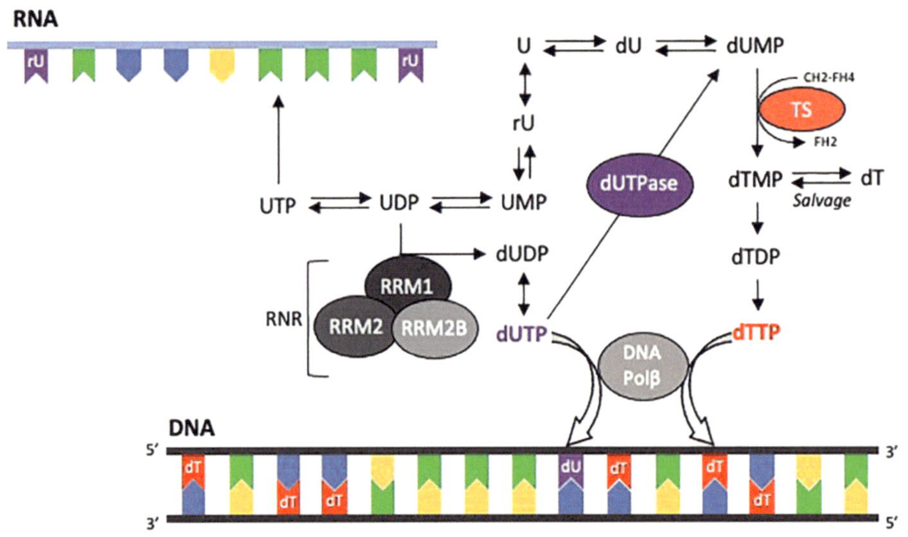

Figure 1.
Uracil biosynthesis and incorporation into genomic RNA and DNA. A simplified schematic showing how uracil (U, purple) and thymidine (T, red) are incorporated into DNA. Normally, uracil is metabolised to UDP then UTP, allowing it to be incorporated into RNA. UDP can also be processed by ribonucleotide reductase (RNR, composed of RRM1/2/2B subunits) to dUDP, which is further metabolised to dUTP. Cells have evolved a system where dUTP levels are kept low by dUTPase converting it into dUMP, which is a substrate for dTTP production. This maintains a high cellular dTTP:dUTP ratio, ensuring minimal uracil misincorporation into DNA since DNA polymerase has similar affinities for dTTP and dUTP. Arrows indicate the direction of a metabolic reaction by an enzyme, double ended arrows indicate a single enzyme can perform a metabolic reaction in both directions. Abbreviations: U = uracil, rU = uridine, dU = deoxyuridine, (d)UMP = (deoxy)uridine monophosphate, (d)UDP = (deoxy)uridine diphosphate, (d)UTP = (deoxy)uridine triphosphate, dT = deoxythymidine, (d) TMP = (deoxy)thymidine monophosphate, (d)TDP = (deoxy)thymidine diphosphate, (d)TTP = (deoxy) thymidine triphosphate, CH2-FH4 = 5,10-methylenetetrahydrofolate, FH2 = dihydrofolate, DNA Polβ = DNA polymerase β, RNR = ribonucleotide reductase, and dUTPase = dUTP nucleotidohydrolase.

4. Uracil

Uracil is a base analogue of thymine and is found in both DNA and RNA (**Figure 1**). As a pyrimidine nucleotide it has an amino acid group at the 2′ position and a carboxy group at the 5′ position. U and T are equivalent in their information storage, transmission and their base pairing with adenine.

In DNA, U is present in pyrimidine dimers, tri- and tetradiphosphate conjugates, DNA repair intermediates and DNA damage-based U incorporation. It is classified as an antimetabolite, which means it can block enzymes that participate in cellular metabolism, where its incorporation into DNA has several biological and pharmacological effects.

Uracil's presence in DNA has been identified to be an important key intermediate in both adaptive and innate immunity (see Section 4.2). In adaptive immunity, U is introduced into DNA by the enzyme activation-induced deaminase (AID), where in B lymphocytes its presence modulates the antibody binding site or initiation of Ig isotype switching [29, 30]. In innate immunity, U in DNA serves as an intermediate in the restriction of viral pathogens with the assistance of the family of APOBEC polynucleotide deaminases, where there is a C:U hypermutation of the viral genome leading to its degradation [31].

Beyond these positive immunity roles of U in DNA, the DNA incorporation of U can negatively impact the cellular functionality of the genetic information storage system, destabilize the Watson-Crick DNA helical structure, inhibit DNA replication, cell growth and development, highlighting the importance of cellular mechanisms to detect and remove inappropriate uracil from DNA.

4.1 Modifications to uracil

Of all the bases, U is the most modified in RNA [32, 33], while in DNA, U has been reported to undergo modifications including methylation [32], hydroxymethylation [34] and oxidation [35]. Methylation, the addition of a methyl group to the nitrogen atom in the ring structure of uracil, can occur at several sites on the base, including the N1 and N3 positions [32]. Hydroxymethylation, the addition of a hydroxymethyl group to the N3 position, is a common modification [32, 35]. Oxidation can also lead to the formation of several different uracil derivates, such as 5-hydroxymethyluracil and 5-formyluracil [35]. Other less prevalent modifications may include glutathionylation, nitration or phosphorylation [36]. These modifications can affect the stability and function of the DNA molecule and may also play a role in regulating gene expression and the development of diseases such as cancer [37, 38].

4.2 Maintenance of uracil-free DNA uracil

Hydrolytic depurination produces about 10,000 abasic sites per cell per day, while hydrolytic deamination of cytosines produces 70–200 uracil bases per day in DNA [13]. The inappropriate U is recognized by family of human UDGs, which cleaves the N-glycosidic bond and thereby generates an abasic sites in the DNA, which are themselves cytotoxic and potentially mutagenic [39]. As mentioned in Section 2, U can arise in DNA either by C deamination or by U mis-incorporation. Deamination of C to U is always mutagenic, if not corrected, as U:G mismatches always leads to C→T or G→A transitions during DNA synthesis and is, interestingly, the most frequent spontaneous mutation of cells, and often found in human tumours. On the other hand, misincorporation of U should not lead to a mutation during DNA synthesis, since U:A pairs would lead to T:A pairs; however, DNA repair mechanisms can be error-prone and, therefore, it is best for the cell to avoid U DNA misincorporation from the onset, as discussed in Section 2.

In almost all the organisms, the nucleotide pools are essential for the correct DNA replication and U is one of the most frequently occurring error bases in DNA; different strategies for "keeping free" the organism of unbalanced levels of nucleotides exists [22]. In this direction, four superfamilies of NTP (nucleoside triphosphate) pyrophosphatases including the nudix hydrolases, trimeric dUTPase, inosine triphosphate pyrophosphatases (ITPases) and all α NTP pyrophosphatases function to hydrolyze the α-β phosphodiester bond of (d)NTPs to monophosphate and pyrophosphoric acid (PPi) focussing on the non-canonical NTPs [22, 23]. The deoxycytidine triphosphatase (dCTPase) and dUTPase are the two main nucleotide hydrolases involved in the elimination of non-canonical nucleotides [22, 24].

The most important mechanisms to maintain U-free-DNA are dUTPase and UDGs [40–42].

4.2.1 dUTPase

The function of dUTPase is to hydrolyze dUTP to dUMP and pyrophosphate, providing a dUMP precursor for the dTMP synthesis, maintaining the balanced dUTP/dTTP ratio and ultimately DNA integrity [43]; this reaction facilitates the cells avoidance of dUTP DNA misincorporation by DNA polymerases during replication (**Figure 1**) [44].

Two distinct protein isoforms of dUTPase, one nuclear and the other mitochondrial, in human cells have been reported [45]. Nuclear dUTPase (DUT-N) and mitochondrial dUTPase (DUT-M) are encoded by two distinct mRNA species of 1.1 and 1.4 kilobases respectively, nonetheless, the dUTPase gene (*DUT*) encode both nuclear and mitochondrial isoforms and arise to mature form by splicing process using different exon patterns [46].

In normal cells, the expression of dUTPase varies, where fluctuations in expression are dependent upon the current state of the cell cycle. Stimulation from mitogenic signals to initiate mitosis triggers the cell to progress from the resting G_0-phase into G_1/S-phase [47]. It is during S-phase of the cell cycle when the DUT-N is increased to provide the dUMP substrate required for dTMP synthesis and subsequent deoxythymidine triphosphate (dTTP) for incorporation into newly synthesized DNA [48]. Overall, the specific activity is over 16,000 nmol of dUMP hydrolyzed per min/mg of dUTPase [49].

4.2.2 Base excision repair

There are four UDGs present in mammalian cells: UNG, SMUG1, TDG and MBD4 [50] that function to recognize and remove U from DNA. This family of enzymes provides redundancy which may be required for specific circumstances and highlights the importance of this repair process. UNG remains central to the repair of U:A misincorporated uracil, whereas all family members are involved in the U:G repair [29].

The process of uracil repair produces an abasic sites, which forms part of Base Excision Repair (BER) pathway in humans, a process that repairs small, non-helix distorting base lesions in the genome [51]. Briefly, a UDG detects U within DNA and 'flips' it out of the double-helix and cleaves the U leaving an abasic site. An AP-endonuclease (APE) then cleaves the DNA-backbone 5′ of the abasic site, creating a single-strand break [52]. During short-patch BER, DNA polymerase β (POLβ) inserts the correct nucleotide into the abasic site and has lyase activity that removes the deoxyribosephosphate (dRP) left over from the abasic site [53]. The open 3′ end (that is left over after DNA polymerase activity) can then be sealed by DNA ligase III (LIG3) and its co-factor XRCC1, removing what is a single-strand break [54, 55]. Alternatively, during long-patch BER; POLδ, POLε and PCNA inserts multiple nucleotides from the abasic site, displacing the downstream DNA (which also contains dRP at its 5′ end), creating a flap [53]. The flap endonuclease 1 (FEN1) then removes this 5′ flap of DNA [56] and DNA ligase 1 (LIG1) is able to seal the single-strand break in the DNA backbone left after this process [57]. See **Figure 2** for BER schematic.

4.3 Uracil-DNA glycosylases

4.3.1 UNG

In humans, two splice variants of Uracil-N-Glycosylase (UNG) are expressed from its gene (*UNG*), with both isoforms containing an identical sequence except for their N-terminal which is unique to each protein. UDG/UNG are interchangeably used to refer to this protein; however, in this text we will refer to the protein as UNG and the

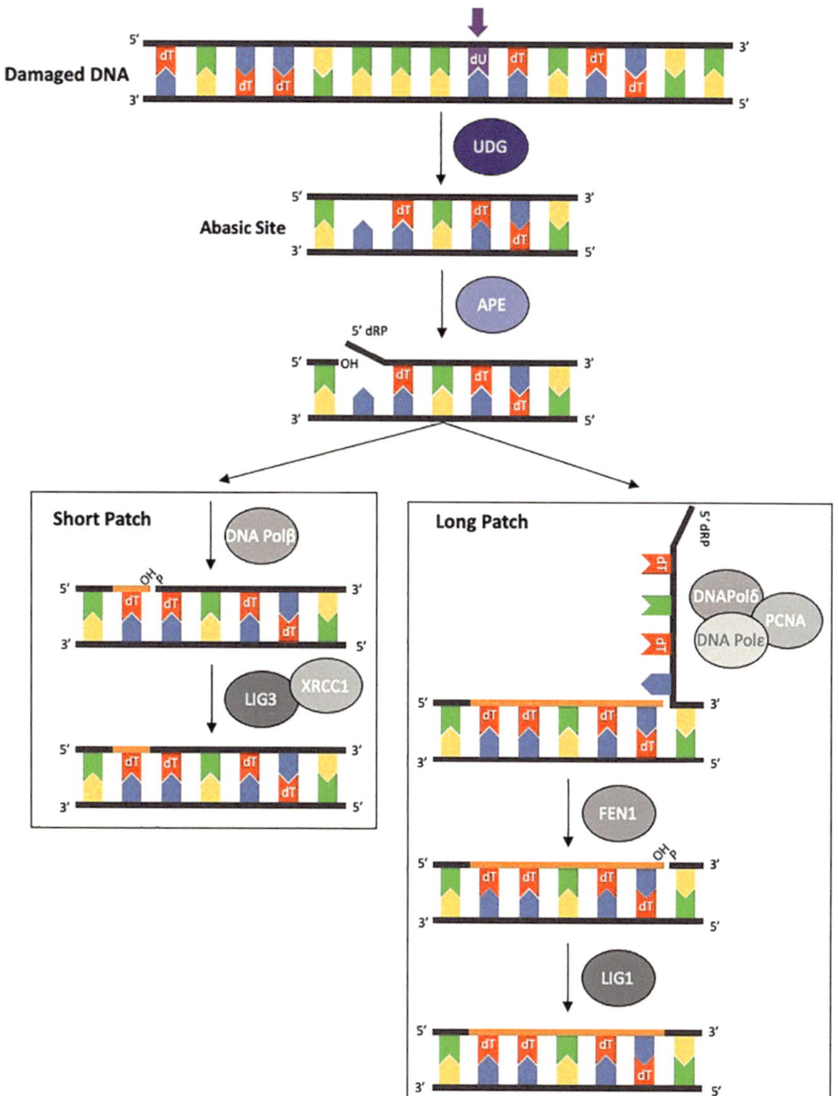

Figure 2.
Detection and removal of uracil in DNA by base excision repair pathway. A simplified schematic showing the two arms of the base excision repair (BER) pathway in the repair of uracil that is either misincorporated (dU:dA) or mismatched (dU:dG) in DNA. A uracil DNA glycosylase, UDG/SMUG1/TDG/MBD4 in humans, detects and 'flips' out the uracil base from the DNA and cleaves it, leaving an abasic site. AP endonuclease (APE) then nicks the DNA backbone 5′ to the abasic site, creating a single-strand DNA break. From there, BER pathway will either proceed down the short patch BER or Long patch BER depending on the type of damage, stage of the cell cycle, and cell differentiation state. In short patch BER, DNA Polβ fills in the gap of the abasic site with the correct base and is also cleaves the deoxyribosephosphate (5′ dRP) left over from the abasic site. After DNA polymerisation, a single-strand DNA break is present and is ligated by LIG3:XRCC1. In long patch BER, DNA Polδ:Polε:PCNA inserts multiple bases from the abasic site, creating a 'flap' of single-stranded DNA. FEN1 is able to cleave this flap and LIG1 seals the single-strand DNA break left over from the process. Abbreviations: 5′ dRP = deoxyribosephosphate, dA = deoxyadenine, dG = deoxyguanine, dU = deoxyuridine, dT = deoxythymidine, APE = Apurinc endonuclease, BER = base excision repair, DNA Polβ = DNA polymerase, FEN1 = flap endonuclease 1, LIG = DNA ligase, MBD4 = methyl-CpG-binding domain protein 4, SMUG1 = single-strand selective monofunctional uracil DNA glycosylase, TDG = thymine DNA glycosylase, UDG = uracil DNA glycosylase, and XRCC1 = X-ray repair cross-complementing protein 1.

superfamily encompassing all the uracil-targeting DNA glycosylases will continue to be referred to as UDG. UNG1 is expressed constitutively in the mitochondria, first as a 35 kDa precursor which is then processed at the N-terminal to a 29 kDa protein, and UNG2 is a 36 kDa serine/threonine phosphoprotein located in the nucleus, which maintains its N-terminal sequence. U detection and removal is predominantly carried out by UNG, in human cells, since it has the highest activity with single-stranded (ss)DNA and is very active with double-stranded (ds)DNA compared to the other UDGs present in human cells (SMUG1, TDG and MBD4) [50, 58, 59]. Additionally, UNG has at least 10^{1-3} times higher turnover than the other three human UDGs [50, 59, 60], with UNG2 being the only DNA glycosylase present in the nucleus that is able to remove U:A pairs close to passing replication forks [61, 62], where UNG is mostly located in replication foci during S-phase [59, 61, 63]. Due to the efficiency of UNG compared to the other UDGs in humans, it is thought that UNG is predominantly responsible for removing U:G mismatches [59, 60]; however, this has not been directly reported except of U:G mismatches produced by activation-induced cytosine deaminase (AID), which are critical in the adaptive immune system.

When an infection occurs in humans, our adaptive immune system will try to generate antibodies specifically for that antigen, which will allow the infection to be efficiently cleared out. B lymphocytes are responsible for generating antibodies, but to generate specific antibodies they need a mechanism to induce heterogeneity, which is achieved via somatic hypermutation (SHM) and class switch recombination (CSR) [29]. The *Ig* loci produces the heavy chain of an antibody and codes for the Ig variable region (produces part of heavy chain that directly binds to antigen) and the Ig constant region (determines class of antibody, which could be IgM, IgG, IgA or IgE). AID deaminates Cs in specific regions of this loci [31]. During CSR, UNG2 targets U and, with APE, generates abasic sites with single-strand breaks. Since AID generates clustered regions of U-containing DNA, this can produce double-strand breaks once UNG2 and AP endonuclease have processed enough of them. This then triggers non-homologous end joining and connects the Ig variable region to a new constant region and determines the class of the antibody. During SHM, AID introduces U into Ig variable region and UNG2 removes these producing abasic sites and error prone polymerases then introduce mutations and alter the DNA sequence. Overall, this means various B lymphocytes produce unique antibodies coded from their *Ig* loci. The unique antibody is exposed on the surface of the B lympocyte and if that antibody has affinity to the antigen presented to it, it will survive and produce Plasma cells, which produce the cloned antibody and then allow the adaptive immune system to target the antigen [64].

In addition to UNG's role in the adaptive immune system, UNG is also involved in the innate immune system. Virally infected cells are exposed to proviral DNA (viral DNA that is yet to become active), which will allow the virus to propagate further by hijacking cellular functions. To counteract this, cells express APOBEC3 enzymes (another DNA cytosine deaminase) that can associate with proviral DNA, before it integrates into the cell's genome, and proceeds to deaminate C→U [65]. This then either leads to degradation of the proviral DNA (with the help of AP endonuclease) or if the proviral DNA does integrate within the genome of the host it is hypermutated (G:C→A:T) and, therefore, non-functional. Other functions of UNG may also include removal of some oxidative products of C including alloxan, isodialuric acid and 5-hydroxyuracil; but it is unknown if this is true *in vivo* [66]. Additionally, UNG2 might be involved in TET-mediated demethylation of cytosine, which would reverse the epigenetic silencing of certain genes [67].

4.3.2 SMUG1

Single-strand-selective Monofunctional Uracil-DNA Glycosylase (SMUG1) was named so because it was originally thought to prefer ssDNA to dsDNA as a substrate [68]; however, it was later found to be specific for dsDNA [60]. SMUG1 is expressed as a 30 kDa protein and is evenly distributed in the nucleus, accumulates in nucleoli and is also found in the cytosol [59]; additionally, unlike the *UNG* gene, the *SMUG1* gene is not regulated by the cell cycle [69]. Like UNG, SMUG1's substrate specificity is greater for U:G mismatches than U:A pairs; however, the catalytic activity of SMUG1 is slower than UNG's [59]. While SMUG1 has been thought to act as a backup to UNG in SHM and CSR in mice, it is worth noting that mice express higher levels of SMUG1 (relative to UNG) than humans do and that UNG/SMUG1 have different roles in initiating BER in mice vs. humans [60, 70]. In addition to its role as a UDG, SMUG1 is the major DNA glycosylase in removing hydroxymethyluracil (5-hmU, an epigenetic modification [71]) from DNA [59, 72–74], with UNG seemingly not having any significant involvement [75].

4.3.3 TDG

Thymine DNA Glycosylase (TDG) is a 46 kDa protein that is located in the nucleus and plasma membrane of the cell. Despite UNG, SMUG1 and TDG sharing less than 10% amino acid similarity they all have similar structures and are located on the same arm of chromosome 12; additionally, they all may have evolved from the same ancestral gene [76]. In contrast to UNG, TDG is highly expressed during G1 and G2-M phases of the cell cycle and not in S-phase, while UNG is highly expressed only in S-phase [77]. TDG is known to remove U:G and T:G mismatches (derived from deaminated 5-methylcytosine (5-mC)) from DNA, with better efficiency with U:G mismatches [78]; however, seems to overall have a very slow turnover rate. Additionally, TDG has higher affinity for U:G mismatches, but also has a very high affinity for abasic sites opposite Gs [79] and it has been reported that TDG SUMOylation helps dissociate it from abasic sites [80]. TDG is also able to remove 5-hmU, thymine glycol halogenated pyrimidines and εC (caused by lipid peroxidation) when they are paired with G. Unlike UNG and SMUG1, when TDG is knocked out of mice it is embryonically lethal [81]. Rather than associating the lethality with TDG's U-DNA glycosylase activity, it is thought this is due to disruption of TDG's association with promoters, transcription factors, transcriptional coactivators and DNA methyltransferase which impairs the epigenetic regulation of developmental genes [81, 82]. Furthermore, TDG has been reported to directly induce DNA demethylation by removing 5-formylC (5-fC) and 5-carboxyC (5-aC) (both derived from TET-mediated oxidation of 5-mC), which leads to BER and repair of the site a non-modified C [83, 84].

4.3.4 MBD4

Methyl-CpG Binding Domain 4 DNA glycosylase (MBD4) is a 66 kDa protein that is predominantly found in the nucleus of the cell. While UNG, SMUG1 and TDG have a similar structure to one another, MBD4 has a N-terminal methyl-binding domain (MBD) which is connected to the C-terminal glycosylase domain that, additionally, has a different structural fold to the other 3 UDGs [85]. However, similar to TDG, MBD4 is able to remove U, T, 5-hmU thymine glycol halogenated pyrimidines and εC when they are paired with G, and MBD4 is not regulated by the cell cycle, the same as SMUG1 [69]. SMUG1's DNA glycosylase activity might predominantly occur near CpG sites since mice with MBD4 knocked out had an increase in C→T transition mutations at CpG sites (DNA methylation sites) [86, 87]. MBD4 has also been reported to have additional roles in apoptosis, transcriptional regulation and active demethylation [82].

4.4 UNG vs. SMUG1 vs. mismatch repair

While UNG seems to be the predominant UDG in removing genomic U, it does not appear to be essential in the overall process. SMUG1 knockout mice's organs had no increase in genomic U, while UNG knockout mice's organs had a 1.9–2.2-fold increase [75]. However, a UNG/SMUG1 double knockout a much greater increase, especially in the liver (25-fold increase), suggesting that while SMUG1 cannot fully compensate for UNG loss it is able to act as a backup [75]. Surprisingly, mice and humans deficient in UNG induce issues related to immunity like problems with CSR and inducing lymphoid hyperplasia [88–91]; however, UNG/SMUG1 single and double knockout mice do not have reduced one-year survival rates [72]. This would suggest that cells can tolerate U, to a certain level at least, and that the major issues that arise from UNG loss seem to be immune-related, likely due to its importance in the adaptive immune system (as discussed in Section 4.2). Paradoxically, cell death induced by too high a levels of genomic U might be induced by the cell's own DNA repair mechanism that induces ssDNA breaks that could lead to dsDNA breaks that are cytotoxic (similar to the mechanism of CSR), in a cancer setting at least [92]. If this is the case, then that would indicate a significant role for UNG/SMUG1 in inducing the cell death in this setting, rather than the high levels of genomic U.

While UNG/SMUG1 double knockout does not reduce one-year survival rates, a triple knockout including MutS homolog 2 (MSH2), a critical enzyme in the DNA repair mechanism termed Mismatch Repair (MMR) severely reduced survival rates when compared to mice with a single MSH2 knockout [72]. This could suggest that while UNG and SMUG1 are complementary to each other's function in removing genomic U, MMR might act as a last resort when the two proteins are lost; however, it is worth mentioning that MSH2 loss alone significantly decreased one-year survival by itself [72]. Furthermore, UNG/SMUG1/MSH2 triple knockout mice also had an increased chance of cancer development (compared to other knockout combinations), which was mostly lymphoma (maybe due to high C deaminase activity in immune cells via AID), suggesting that these three proteins are key to maintaining genomic stability, potentially via the removal of genomic U [72].

Overall, one could hypothesis that high levels of genomic U, in the acute setting, could lead to cell death induced by the DNA repair machinery not being able repair the damage it inflicts initially for repair; however, if high levels of genomic U occur when UNG/SMUG1/MMR are not present then the cells would not initially die but over time would acquire a high amount of mutations, leading to either death or cancerous phenotypes. Though, a lot more work is needed to validate this hypothesis but visualising cell death in a UNG/SMUG1/MMR deficient cell with high levels of genomic U might reveal some answers.

5. Therapeutic-induced thymine-less death

As mentioned, U:A pairs in DNA arise from dUTP misincorporation by DNA polymerase since they use dTTP and dUTP with similar efficiencies. In fact, several studies have confirmed that DNA-cytosine deaminase or U:G mismatches constitute a major mutational DNA lesion that contributes to various diseases, including cancer development and progression [93]. To counteract uracil in DNA, the cell has evolved the two proteins TS and dUTPase (see Section 4.1), which lowers the dUTP:dTTP ratio and thereby reduces dUTP use by DNA polymerases by having more dTTP available. The first step is by dUTPase, which converts dUTP into dUMP; thus, dUTP levels are decreased and TS's substrate (dUMP) is increased simultaneously. TS then converts dUMP into dTMP by attaching a methyl group to the C5 position of U's aromatic ring, the methyl group being donated by 5,10-methylenetetrahydrofolate (5,10-CH_2THF, a folate derivative). Two extra kinase steps are then needed to convert dTMP into dTTP, which can be readily processed for DNA synthesis.

Originally, it was rationalized that targeting the pyrimidine biosynthesis pathway would be an effective method in treating cancer, based on several findings including the observation that U was specifically incorporated into the nucleic acid fractions of rat tumours [94]. This eventually led to the development of the fluoropyrimidine 5-Fluoruracil (5-FU) in 1957 [95], one of the best know chemotherapies for cancer treatment in modern times. 5-FU's mechanism of action as an anti-cancer therapy seem to be complicated but what is known is that metabolites produced from it can are incorporated into DNA and RNA, which induces cellular stress and then subsequent cell death in cancer cells. Additionally, one of 5-FU's metabolites (FdUMP) is able to inhibit and it is through this method a range of fluoropyrimidines and antifolates (which indirectly inhibit TS) have been designed and used for treatment of large range or cancer types, in which their uses still seem to be growing today [96].

Building on 5-FU's clinical success, several additional cancer therapies such Pemetrexed, Capecitabine, Methotrexate and Raltitrexed were developed and are currently used in cancer chemotherapy regimens to inhibit TS and modify the cancer cell's viability as a consequence of the depletion of dTTP pools, called *thymine less-death*. Thymine less-death results from an imbalance in dUTP/TTP levels, where dTTP is depleted and there is an increase in dUTP, misincorporation of uracil into DNA and following attempted repair results in DNA double-strand breaks (DSB) [97, 98]. To a global understanding of involved mechanism it is important to highlight that the dUMP pools needed for TMP biosynthesis depends on dCMP deamination and UDP reduction by deoxycytidylate deaminase (DCD) and RNR, respectively [39].

6. Conclusions

Uracil, a non-canonical DNA base, has been identified as one of the major bases misincorporated into DNA either through the process of cytosine deamination or through the introduction by DNA polymerase. The presence of uracil in DNA, while important for specific adaptive and innate immune functions, in other contexts threatens genetic stability and continuity, where dysregulated genomic uracil levels has been linked to various disease, including cancer. Several key enzymes have been identified to collaborate in maintaining uracil-free DNA through modulation of uracil levels within the cell by dUTPase, as well as the uracil-DNA glycosylase family (UNG, SMUG1, TDG, MBD4), who function to recognize and excise uracil from DNA, where UNG1 and UNG2 are the most competent and widely used for uracil misincorporation in DNA.

Acknowledgments

We would like to thank the staff, past and present, of the Nucleotide Metabolism Research Group at Queen's University Belfast for their dedication to the research on uracil metabolism. In addition, we would like to thank Dr Peter Wilson and Dr Robert Ladner for their valuable insights into the biology and many valuable conversations that have helped shape the research.

Conflict of interest

The authors declare no conflict of interest.

Nomenclature

5-aC	5-carboxyC
5-fC	5-formylC
5-FU	5-Fluorouracil
5-hmU	Hydroxymethyluracil
A	Adeninie
AID	Activation-induced deaminase
APE	AP-endonuclease
APOBEC	Apolipoprotein B MRNA editing enzyme catalytic subunit
ATP	Adenosine triphosphate
BER	Base exicision repair
C	Cytosine
CSR	Class switch recombination
CTP	Cytosine triphosphate
dCTPase	Deoxycytidine triphosphatase
DNA	Deoxyribonucleic Acid
dNTPs	Deoxynucleotide triphosphosphates
dRP	Deoxyribosephosphate
DSB	Double-strand breaks
dTMP	Deoxythymidine monophosphate
dTTP	Deoxythymidine triphosphate
dUMP	Deoxyuridine monophosphate
dUTP	Deoxyuridine triphosphate
dUTPase	dUTP nucleotidehydrolase
FEN1	Flap endonuclease 1
G	Guanine
GTP	Guanosine triphosphate
ITPase	Inosine triphosphate pyrophosphatases
LIG3	DNA ligase III
MBD4	Methyl-CpG binding domain 4 DNA glycosylase
MMR	Mismatch repair
mRNA	Messenger RNA
MSH2	MutS homolog 2
NDPK	Nucleoside diphosphate kinase
NTPs	Nucleotide triphosphosphates

PCNA	Proliferating cell nuclear antigen
POLβ	DNA polymerase β
RNA	Ribonucleic Acid
RNR	Ribonucleotide reductase
SHM	Somatic hypermutation
SMUG1	Single-strand-selective monofunctional uracil-DNA glycosylase
T	Thymine
TDG	Thymine DNA glycosylase
tRNA	Transfer RNA
TS	Thymidylate synthase
U	Uracil
UDG	Uracil-DNA glycosylase
UNG	Uracil-N-Glycosylase
UTP	Uracil triphosphate

Author details

Jamie Z. Roberts and Melissa J. LaBonte*
Patrick G Johnston Centre for Cancer Research, Queen's University Belfast, Belfast, United Kingdom

*Address all correspondence to: m.labontewilson@qub.ac.uk

References

[1] Takeda DY, Dutta A. DNA replication and progression through S phase. Oncogene. 2005;**24**:2827-2843

[2] Ganai RA, Johansson E. DNA replication—AMatter of Fidelity. Molecular Cell. 2016;**62**:745-755

[3] Fragkos M, Ganier O, Coulombe P, et al. DNA replication origin activation in space and time. Nature Reviews. Molecular Cell Biology. 2015;**16**:360-374

[4] Hanahan D, Weinberg RA. The hallmarks of cancer. Cell. 2000;**100**:57-70

[5] Hanahan D, Weinberg RA. Hallmarks of cancer: The next generation. Cell. 2011;**144**:646-674

[6] Jiricny J. Replication errors: Cha(lle) nging the genome. The EMBO Journal. 1998;**17**:6427-6436

[7] Pizzarello S, Shock E. The organic composition of carbonaceous meteorites: The evolutionary story ahead of biochemistry. Cold Spring Harbor Perspectives in Biology. 2010;**2**:a002105

[8] Costanzo G, Saladino R, Crestini C, et al. Formamide as the main building block in the origin of nucleic acids. BMC Evolutionary Biology. 2007;**7**:1-8

[9] Ferusa M, Nesvorný D, Šponer J, et al. High-energy chemistry of formamide: A unified mechanism of nucleobase formation. Proceedings of the National Academy of Sciences of the United States of America. 2015;**112**:657-662

[10] Šponer JE, Šponer J, Nováková O, et al. Emergence of the first catalytic oligonucleotides in a Formamide-based origin scenario. Chemistry. 2016;**22**:3572-3586

[11] Saladino R, Carota E, Botta G, et al. Meteorite-catalyzed syntheses of nucleosides and of other prebiotic compounds from formamide under proton irradiation. Proceedings of the National Academy of Sciences of the United States of America. 2015;**112**:E2746-E2755

[12] Saladino R, Botta G, Delfino M, et al. Meteorites as catalysts for prebiotic chemistry. Chemistry—A European Journal. 2013;**19**:16916-16922

[13] Lindahl T. Instability and decay of the primary structure of DNA. Nature. 1993;**362**:709-715

[14] Lindahl T. Irreversible heat inactivation of transfer ribonucleic acids. Journal of Biological Chemistry. 1967;**242**:1970-1973

[15] Singer B, Fraenkel-Conrat H. The nature of the breaks occurring in TMV-RNA under various conditions. Biochimica et Biophysica Acta. 1963;**76**:143-145

[16] Leu K, Obermayer B, Rajamani S, et al. The prebiotic evolutionary advantage of transferring genetic information from RNA to DNA. Nucleic Acids Research. 2011;**39**:8135-8147

[17] Flanegan JB, Greenberg GR. Regulation of deoxyribonucleotide biosynthesis during in vivo bacteriophage T4 DNA replication. Intrinsic control of synthesis of thymine and 5-hydroxymethylcytosine deoxyribonucleotides at precise ratio found in DNA. Journal of Biological Chemistry. 1977;**252**:3019-3027

[18] Lundin D, Berggren G, Logan DT, et al. The origin and evolution of ribonucleotide reduction. Life. 2015;**5**:604

[19] Ma W, Yu C, Zhang W, et al. The emergence of DNA in the RNA world: An in silico simulation study of genetic takeover. BMC Evolutionary Biology. 2015;**15**:1-16

[20] Hofer A, Crona M, Logan DT, et al. DNA building blocks: Keeping control of manufacture. Critical Reviews in Biochemistry and Molecular Biology. 2012;**47**:50-63

[21] Vértessy BG, Tóth J. Keeping uracil out of DNA: Physiological role, structure and catalytic mechanism of dUTPases. Accounts of Chemical Research. 2009;**42**:97

[22] Kerepesi C, Szabó JE, Papp-Kádár V, et al. Life without dUTPase. Frontiers in Microbiology. 2016;**7**:1768

[23] Galperin Y, Moroz OV, Wilson KS, et al. House cleaning, a part of good housekeeping. Molecular Microbiology. 2006;**59**:5-19

[24] Requena CE, Moreno GṔ, Andŕas H, et al. The nucleotidohydrolases DCTPP1 and dUTPase are involved in the cellular response to decitabine. Biochemical Journal. 2016;**473**:2635-2643

[25] Niida H, Shimada M, Murakami H, et al. Mechanisms of dNTP supply that play an essential role in maintaining genome integrity in eukaryotic cells. Cancer Science. 2010;**101**:2505-2509

[26] Kolberg M, Strand KR, Graff P, et al. Structure, function, and mechanism of ribonucleotide reductases. Biochim Biophys Acta Proteins Proteom. 2004;**1699**:1-34

[27] Aye Y, Li M, Long MJC, et al. Ribonucleotide reductase and cancer: Biological mechanisms and targeted therapies. Oncogene. 2015;**34**:2011-2021

[28] Mathews CK. Deoxyribonucleotide metabolism, mutagenesis and cancer. Nature Reviews Cancer. 2015;**15**:528-539

[29] Visnes T, Doseth B, Pettersen HS, et al. Uracil in DNA and its processing by different DNA glycosylases. Philosophical Transactions of the Royal Society B: Biological Sciences. 2009;**364**:563

[30] Safavi S, Larouche A, Zahn A, et al. The uracil-DNA glycosylase UNG protects the fitness of normal and cancer B cells expressing AID. NAR Cancer. 2020;**2**:zcaa019

[31] Çakan E, Gunaydin G. Activation induced cytidine deaminase: An old friend with new faces. Frontiers in Immunology. 2022;**13**:965312

[32] Mishanina T, v., Koehn EM, Kohen A. Mechanisms and inhibition of uracil methylating enzymes. Bioorganic Chemistry. 2012;**43**:37

[33] Sheng J, Zhang W, Hassan AEA, et al. Hydrogen bond formation between the naturally modified nucleobase and phosphate backbone. Nucleic Acids Research. 2012;**40**:8111

[34] Pfaffeneder T, Spada F, Wagner M, et al. Tet oxidizes thymine to 5-hydroxymethyluracil in mouse embryonic stem cell DNA. Nature Chemical Biology. 2014;**10**:574-581

[35] Masaoka A, Terato H, Kobayashi M, et al. Oxidation of thymine to 5-Formyluracil in DNA promotes Misincorporation of dGMP and subsequent elongation of a mismatched primer terminus by DNA polymerase. Journal of Biological Chemistry. 2001;**276**:16501-16510

[36] Jha JS, Yin J, Haldar T, et al. Reconsidering the chemical Nature

of Strand breaks derived from Abasic sites in cellular DNA: Evidence for 3′-Glutathionylation. Journal of the American Chemical Society. 2022;**144**:10471-10482

[37] Carr CE, Khutsishvili I, Gold B, et al. Thermodynamic stability of DNA duplexes comprising the simplest T → du substitutions. Biochemistry. 2018;**57**:5666-5671

[38] Hofer A, Liu ZJ, Balasubramanian S. Detection, structure and function of modified DNA bases. Journal of the American Chemical Society. 2019;**141**:6420-6429

[39] Lindahl T. An N-glycosidase from Escherichia coli that releases free uracil from DNA containing deaminated cytosine residues. Proceedings of the National Academy of Sciences of the United States of America. 1974;**71**:3649-3653

[40] Castillo-Acosta VM, Aguilar-Pereyra F, Vidal AE, et al. Trypanosomes lacking uracil-DNA glycosylase are hypersensitive to antifolates and present a mutator phenotype. International Journal of Biochemistry and Cell Biology. 2012;**44**:1555-1568

[41] Pecsi I, Hirmondo R, Brown AC, et al. The dutpase enzyme is essential in mycobacterium smegmatis. PLoS One. 2012;**7**:e37461

[42] Kerepesi C, Szabó JE, Grolmusz V, et al. Life without dUTPase. Frontiers in Microbiology. 2016;**7**:1768

[43] Mol CD, Harris JM, McIntosh EM, et al. Human dUTP pyrophosphatase: Uracil recognition by a β hairpin and active sites formed by three separate subunits. Structure. 1996;**4**:1077-1092

[44] Tinkelenberg BA, Fazzone W, Lynch FJ, et al. Identification of sequence determinants of human nuclear dUTPase isoform localization. Experimental Cell Research. 2003;**287**:39-46

[45] Ladner RD, McNulty DE, Carr SA, et al. Characterization of distinct nuclear and mitochondrial forms of human deoxyuridine triphosphate nucleotidohydrolase. The Journal of Biological Chemistry. 1996;**271**:7745-7751

[46] Ladner RD, Caradonna SJ. The human dUTPase gene encodes both nuclear and mitochondrial isoforms. Differential expression of the isoforms and characterization of a cDNA encoding the mitochondrial species. The Journal of Biological Chemistry. 1997;**272**:19072-19080

[47] Malumbres M, Barbacid M. To cycle or not to cycle: A critical decision in cancer. Nature Reviews. Cancer. 2001;**1**:222-231

[48] Lane AN, Fan TWM. Regulation of mammalian nucleotide metabolism and biosynthesis. Nucleic Acids Research. 2015;**43**:2466-2485

[49] Caradonna SJ, Adamkiewicz DM. Purification and properties of the deoxyuridine triphosphate nucleotidohydrolase enzyme derived from HeLa S3 cells. Comparison to a distinct dUTP nucleotidohydrolase induced in herpes simplex virus-infected HeLa S3 cells. Journal of Biological Chemistry. 1984;**259**:5459-5464

[50] Krokan HE, Drabløs F, Slupphaug G. Uracil in DNA—Occurrence, consequences and repair. Oncogene. 2002;**21**:8935-8948

[51] Wallace SS. Base excision repair: A critical player in many games. DNA Repair (Amst). 2014;**19**:14

[52] Hadi SM, Goldthwait DA. Endonuclease II of *Escherichia coli*.

Degradation of partially Depurinated deoxyribonucleic acid. Biochemistry. 1971;**10**:4986-4994

[53] Beard WA, Prasad R, Wilson SH. Activities and mechanism of DNA polymerase β. Methods in Enzymology. 2006;**408**:91-107

[54] Caldecott KW, Tucker JD, Stanker LH, et al. Characterization of the XRCC1-DNA ligase III complex in vitro and its absence from mutant hamster cells. Nucleic Acids Research. 1995;**23**:4836-4843

[55] Cappelli E, Taylor R, Cevasco M, et al. Involvement of XRCC1 and DNA ligase III gene products in DNA Base excision repair. Journal of Biological Chemistry. 1997;**272**:23970-23975

[56] Kao HI, Henricksen LA, Liu Y, et al. Cleavage specificity of Saccharomyces cerevisiae flap endonuclease 1 suggests a double-flap structure as the cellular substrate. Journal of Biological Chemistry. 2002;**277**:14379-14389

[57] Pascucci B, Stucki M, Jónsson ZO, et al. Long Patch Base excision repair with purified human proteins: DNA Ligase I as patch size mediator for DNA polymerases δ and ε. Journal of Biological Chemistry. 1999;**274**:33696-33702

[58] Krokan H, Urs WC. Uracil DNa-glycosylase from HeLa cells: General properties, substrate specificity and effect of uracil analogs. Nucleic Acids Research. 1981;**9**:2599-2614

[59] Kavli B, Sundheim O, Akbari M, et al. hUNG2 is the major repair enzyme for removal of uracil from U: A matches, U:G mismatches, and U in single-stranded DNA, with hSMUG1 as a broad specificity backup. The Journal of Biological Chemistry. 2002;**277**:39926-39936

[60] Doseth B, Visnes T, Wallenius A, et al. Uracil-DNA glycosylase in base excision repair and adaptive immunity: Species differences between man and mouse. The Journal of Biological Chemistry. 2011;**286**:16669-16680

[61] Otterlei M, Warbrick E, Nagelhus TA, et al. Post-replicative base excision repair in replication foci. The EMBO Journal. 1999;**18**:3834

[62] Nilsen H, Rosewell I, Robins P, et al. Uracil-DNA glycosylase (UNG)-deficient mice reveal a primary role of the enzyme during DNA replication. Molecular Cell. 2000;**5**:1059-1065

[63] Hagen L, Kavli B, Sousa MML, et al. Cell cycle-specific UNG2 phosphorylations regulate protein turnover, activity and association with RPA. The EMBO Journal. 2008;**27**:51-61

[64] di Noia J, Neuberger MS. Altering the pathway of immunoglobulin hypermutation by inhibiting uracil-DNA glycosylase. Nature. 2002;**419**:43-48

[65] Wong L, Sami A, Chelico L. Competition for DNA binding between the genome protector replication protein A and the genome modifying APOBEC3 single-stranded DNA deaminases. Nucleic Acids Research. 2022;**50**:12039-12057

[66] Dizdaroglu M, Karakaya A, Jaruga P, et al. Novel activities of human uracil DNA N-glycosylase for cytosine-derived products of oxidative DNA damage. Nucleic Acids Research. 1996;**24**:418-422

[67] Xue JH, Xu GF, Gu TP, et al. Uracil-DNA glycosylase UNG promotes Tet-mediated DNA demethylation. The Journal of Biological Chemistry. 2016;**291**:731

[68] Haushalter KA, Stukenberg PT, Kirschner MW, et al. Identification of a new uracil-DNA glycosylase

family by expression cloning using synthetic inhibitors. Current Biology. 1999;**9**:174-185

[69] Mjelle R, Hegre SA, Aas PA, et al. Cell cycle regulation of human DNA repair and chromatin remodeling genes. DNA Repair (Amst). 2015;**30**:53-67

[70] Nilsen H, Haushalter KA, Robins P, et al. Excision of deaminated cytosine from the vertebrate genome: Role of the SMUG1 uracil–DNA glycosylase. The EMBO Journal. 2001;**20**:4278

[71] Kawasaki F, Beraldi D, Hardisty RE, et al. Genome-wide mapping of 5-hydroxymethyluracil in the eukaryote parasite Leishmania. Genome Biology. 2017;**18**:1-8

[72] Kemmerich K, Dingler FA, Rada C, et al. Germline ablation of SMUG1 DNA glycosylase causes loss of 5-hydroxymethyluracil- and UNG-backup uracil-excision activities and increases cancer predisposition of Ung−/−Msh2−/− mice. Nucleic Acids Research. 2012;**40**:6016

[73] Boorstein RJ, Cummings A, Marenstein DR, et al. Definitive identification of mammalian 5-hydroxymethyluracil DNA N-glycosylase activity as SMUG1. The Journal of Biological Chemistry. 2001;**276**:41991-41997

[74] Pettersen HS, Visnes T, Vågbø CB, et al. UNG-initiated base excision repair is the major repair route for 5-fluorouracil in DNA, but 5-fluorouracil cytotoxicity depends mainly on RNA incorporation. Nucleic Acids Research. 2011;**39**:8430-8444

[75] Alsøe L, Sarno A, Carracedo S, et al. Uracil accumulation and mutagenesis dominated by cytosine deamination in CpG dinucleotides in mice lacking UNG and SMUG1. Scientific Reports. 2017;**7**:7199

[76] Pearl LH. Structure and function in the uracil-DNA glycosylase superfamily. Mutation Research—DNA Repair. 2000;**460**:165-181

[77] Hardeland U, Kunz C, Focke F, et al. Cell cycle regulation as a mechanism for functional separation of the apparently redundant uracil DNA glycosylases TDG and UNG2. Nucleic Acids Research. 2007;**35**:3859-3867

[78] Gallinari P, Jiricny J. A new class of uracil-DNA glycosylases related to human thymine-DNA glycosylase. Nature. 1996;**383**:735-738

[79] Hardeland U, Bentele M, Lettieri T, et al. Thymine DNA glycosylase. Progress in Nucleic Acid Research and Molecular Biology. 2001;**68**:235-253

[80] Baba D, Maita N, Jee JG, et al. Crystal structure of thymine DNA glycosylase conjugated to SUMO-1. Nature. 2005;**435**:979-982

[81] Cortázar D, Kunz C, Selfridge J, et al. Embryonic lethal phenotype reveals a function of TDG in maintaining epigenetic stability. Nature. 2011;**470**:419-423

[82] Sjolund AB, Senejani AG, Sweasy JB. MBD4 and TDG: Multifaceted DNA glycosylases with ever expanding biological roles. Mutation Research. 2013;**743-744**:12-25

[83] Maiti A, Drohat AC. Thymine DNA glycosylase can rapidly excise 5-formylcytosine and 5-carboxylcytosine: Potential implications for active demethylation of CpG sites. The Journal of Biological Chemistry. 2011;**286**:35334-35338

[84] He YF, Li BZ, Li Z, et al. Tet-mediated formation of 5-carboxylcytosine and its excision by TDG in mammalian DNA. Science. 2011;**333**:1303-1307

[85] Wu P, Qiu C, Sohail A, et al. Mismatch repair in methylated DNA. Structure and activity of the mismatch-specific thymine glycosylase domain of methyl-CpG-binding protein MBD4. The Journal of Biological Chemistry. 2003;**278**:5285-5291

[86] Wong E, Yang K, Kuraguchi M, et al. Mbd4 inactivation increases Cright-arrowT transition mutations and promotes gastrointestinal tumor formation. Proceedings of the National Academy of Sciences of the United States of America. 2002;**99**:14937-14942

[87] Millar CB, Guy J, Sansom OJ, et al. Enhanced CpG mutability and tumorigenesis in MBD4-deficient mice. Science. 2002;**297**:403-405

[88] Imai K, Slupphaug G, Lee WI, et al. Human uracil-DNA glycosylase deficiency associated with profoundly impaired immunoglobulin class-switch recombination. Nature Immunology. 2003;**4**:1023-1028

[89] Rada C, Williams GT, Nilsen H, et al. Immunoglobulin isotype switching is inhibited and somatic hypermutation perturbed in UNG-deficient mice. Current Biology. 2002;**12**:1748-1755

[90] Andersen S, Ericsson M, Dai HY, et al. Monoclonal B-cell hyperplasia and leukocyte imbalance precede development of B-cell malignancies in uracil-DNA glycosylase deficient mice. DNA Repair (Amst). 2005;**4**:1432-1441

[91] Nilsen H, Stamp G, Andersen S, et al. Gene-targeted mice lacking the Ung uracil-DNA glycosylase develop B-cell lymphomas. Oncogene. 2003;**22**: 5381-5386

[92] Davison C, Morelli R, Knowlson C, et al. Targeting nucleotide metabolism enhances the efficacy of anthracyclines and anti-metabolites in triple-negative breast cancer. NPJ Breast Cancer. 2021;**7**:38

[93] Krokan HE, Sætrom P, Aas PA, et al. Error-free versus mutagenic processing of genomic uracil—Relevance to cancer. DNA Repair (Amst). 2014;**19**:38-47

[94] Rutman R, Cantarow A, Paschkis AE. Studies in 2-Acetylaminofluorene Carcinogenesis III. The Utilization of Uracil-2-C14 by Preneoplastic Rat Liver and Rat Hepatoma*. Cancer Research. 1954;**14**:119-123

[95] Heidelberger C, Chaudhuri NK, Danneberg P, et al. Fluorinated pyrimidines: A new class of tumour-inhibitory compounds. Nature. 1957;**179**:663-666

[96] Wilson PM, Danenberg PV, Johnston PG, et al. Standing the test of time: Targeting thymidylate biosynthesis in cancer therapy. Nature Reviews Clinical Oncology. 2014;**11**:282-298

[97] Martín CM, Guzmán EC. DNA replication initiation as a key element in thymineless death. DNA Repair (Amst). 2011;**10**:94-101

[98] Webley SD, Welsh SJ, Jackman AL, et al. The ability to accumulate deoxyuridine triphosphate and cellular response to thymidylate synthase (TS) inhibition. British Journal of Cancer. 2001;**85**:446-452

Chapter 3

Modified (2′,5′)Oligonucleotides: The Influence of Structural and Steriochemical Factors on Biological and Immunotropic Activity

Elena Kalinichenko

Abstract

The synthesis of a large number of analogs of natural 2-5A and the results of studies to clarify the relationship between the structure and spatial organization (stereochemistry) and the biological properties of analogs 2-5A have convincingly demonstrated that by changing the structure and/or stereochemistry of molecules, it is possible to achieve either strengthening of known properties or giving new ones. The replacement of the adenosine fragment with 1-deazaadenosine (c^1A) or 3-deazaadenosine (c^3A) at various positions of the 2-5A chain demonstrated the role of each of the nitrogen atoms of the adenine heterocycle in the processes of binding and activation of RNase L. The use of conformationally rigid fluorodeoxyadenylates in enzymatic reactions made it possible to differentiate the role of structural and stereochemical factors and demonstrate the influence of molecules' stereochemistry on their biological properties. Oligomers with *ribo*-[(2′,5′)A_2A_{RA}] and *lixo*-[(2′,5′)A_2A^{LA}] conformation in the (A3) terminal fragment showed activity against diseases associated with disorders of T-cell immunity, autoimmune diseases, viral infections, lymphocytic malignant transformations, prevention of transplant rejection after bone marrow transplantation and, possibly, in the treatment of complications associated with the reaction of the transplanted tissue and the recipient's tissue.

Keywords: 2-5A, (2′,5′)oligoadenylates analogs, RNase L, stereochemistry, NK-cells, lytic activity, phagocytosis, immunosuppressive activity

1. Introduction

(2′,5′)Oligoadenylates represent one of the elements of cellular endogenous antiviral defense which is induced by interferon in response to RNA molecules synthesized in virally infected cells [1, 2]. The key role of 5′-triphosphorylated (2′-5′) oligoadenylates, 2-5A [ppp(A2′p5′)$_n$A, n = 2÷15; mainly, trimer, n = 2] (**Figure 1**), in the antiviral effect of interferon is widely recognized. Oligoadenylates bind and then activate 2-5A-dependent endoribonuclease (RNase L) contributing to the hydrolysis

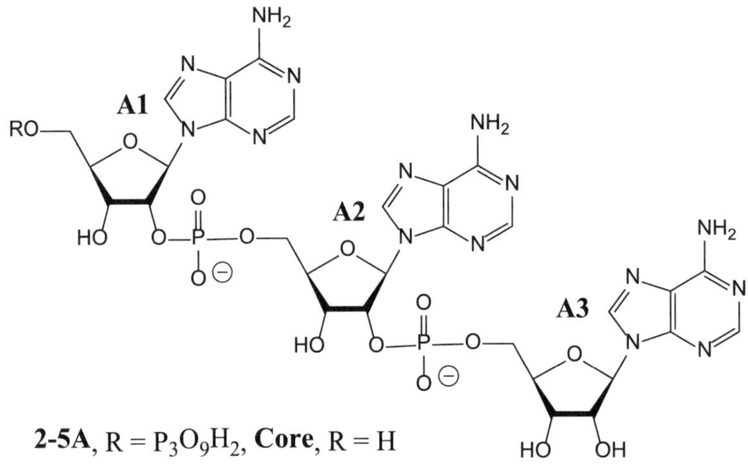

Figure 1.
*Structures of 5′-phosphates of the trimer 2′,5′-oligoadenylic acid [pppA2′p5′A2′p5′A (**2-5A**)] and dephosphorylated analog [**Core**].*

of viral mRNA and, consequently, the inhibition of viral protein synthesis [3–5]. Low molecular weight oligomers are present in nanomolar (10^{-9} M) concentration in living organisms and play a crucial role in the antiviral effects of interferon, maintaining early pregnancy, endochondral ossification, myogenesis, neuronal differentiation, apoptosis, heat-shock response, etc. Findings obtained from biochemical examinations of the cellular endogenous antiviral defense aroused great interest in analyzing of the 2-5A system general functioning mechanisms, as well as biochemical role played by its specific components [6–10].

However, 2-5A is rapidly cleaved by 2′-5′-phosphodiesterase [11, 12]. Moreover, the molecule has a large negative charge and is incapable to penetrate the cell membrane. These shortcomings can be eliminated by modifying the molecule while retaining the ability to bind to RNase L. Modifications can be made to the base, sugar, or phosphate fragments. But the development of new modified oligonucleotides is a challenge due to chemical, electronic, and steric problems. Additionally, the scope of application of oligonucleotides can be expanded through their structure chemical modification. Therefore, synthetic oligonucleotides are currently used for a wide range of purposes including biotechnology, molecular biology, diagnostics, and therapy.

In this review, the main focus will be on ppp(A2′p5′)$_2$A and dephosphorylated trimers modified in the nucleotide part, and the analysis of effects of structural and stereochemical characteristics on some biological properties including immunotropic activity.

2. (2′-5′)Oligoadenylates modified on the heterocyclic base

The contribution of various functional groups of each individual 2-5A nucleoside moiety is highly specific to both RNase L binding and activation. There have been scientific publications in which ppp(A2′p5′)$_2$A or trimer thereof were modified in the nucleotide part and subsequently assessed for their sustained ability to activate endonuclease. As a result of these studies, structural requirements emerged that are important for RNase L activation (reviewed in [4, 13]). Adenine bases were modified in several positions [14, 15], or even substituted by other base moieties [15, 16]. Substitution of H-8 in adenine with a Br atom [17], a methyl group [18], or a hydroxyl group [19] seems to change mainly the base-to-ribose orientation, which may have implications for endonuclease binding capacity. Despite the assumption of minor role of the central adenosine residue [14], its substitution by uridine reduces binding and activation significantly [16]. These studies have generally shown that the presence of adenosine in all positions of the 2-5A chain is crucial for the mediator activity and minimal modifications of heterocyclic bases might be acceptable.

Substitution of the adenosine moiety with 1-deazaadenosine (c^1A) or 3-deazaadenosine (c^3A) at different positions of the 2-5A chain first allowed to establish the role played by each of the adenine heterocycle nitrogen atoms in RNase L binding and activation [20–22].

The 2-5A analogs where adenosine was sequentially substituted by inosine show that (A1) NH_2–C6–N1 moiety of the adenosine residue is critical for binding to RNase L. The same 2′-terminal (A3) adenosine residue moiety is required for the enzyme activation [14]. However, during the examination of the structure/biological activity dependence, a substitution of adenosine by inosine shall be considered as it causes two simultaneous alterations of the chemical structure including the transformation of adenine primary exocyclic 6-amino group into a keto function and the transformation of adenine N1 nitrogen atom into a NH part of hypoxanthine (**Figure 2**). Thus, previous data did not allow us to draw a definite conclusion as to what caused the loss of binding and/or activating ability of the above analogs substituted for inosine—the loss of exocyclic adenosine NH_2-C6 group or transition of the tertiary adenine N1 nitrogen atom to the secondary atom in hypoxanthine? The use of 2-5A 1-deazaadenosine analogs resolved the above ambiguity since the substitution of adenosine by 1-deazaadenosine removes solely the adenine N1 nitrogen atom turning it into a CH moiety yet leaving the exocyclic primary amino function unchanged (**Figure 2**) [20, 21].

The pA(c^1A)A deaza analog containing c^1A in the trimer middle chain link was highly active which is consistent with data on the inosine analog pA(**I**)A activity [14]. Substitution of (A1) moiety with both c^1A, p(c^1A)A_2, and inosine, p(I)A_2 reduces the ability to activate RNase L by about a factor of 33. So the loss of activity is due to the absence of tertiary N1 nitrogen atom and not the absence of the exocyclic amino group. These results are consistent with data provided in [23] which showed that 2-5A

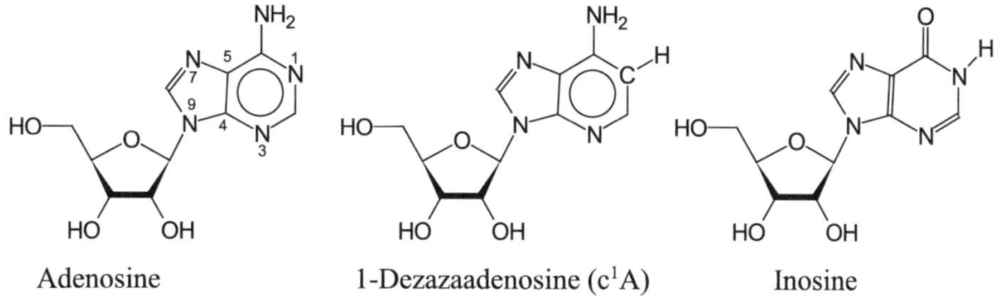

Figure 2.
Structural formulas of adenosine (A), 1-dezazaadenosine (c^1A), and inosine (I).

analog containing 1-(β-D-ribofuranosyl)-1H-1,2,4-triazolo-3-carboxamide (ribavirin) in (A1) moiety activates recombinant RNase L from human CEM cell extracts more effectively compared to the parent trimer. The carboxamide group of ribavirin is probably better in mimicking NH_2–C6–N1 moiety 5′-terminal adenosine compared to c^1A. It should also be noted that N1 of (A1) nitrogen atom of adenosine moiety can be pivotal in binding (2′-5′) oligomers with RNase L. Deazaadenosine analog $pA_2(^1A)$ showed a 20-fold increase in activating ability compared to pA_2(**I**) and as much as a 5-fold decrease compared to the parent tetramer pA_4. Obviously, the NH_2-C6 exocyclic amino group of 2-5A (A3) adenosine moiety is responsible for the conformational "switch" that induces activation of RNase L.

It was shown that substitution of 5′-terminal or 2′-terminal adenosine for c^3A produced respective analogs including p5′(c^3A)2′p5′A2′p5′A and p5′A2′p5′A2′p5′(c^3A) which were not inferior to the parent tetramer in activating RNase L ($EC_{50} \leq 1$ nM) [22]. In contrast, p5′A2′p5′(c^3A)2′p5′A showed a reduced ability to activate RNase L ($EC_{50} \leq 10$ nM). These data are consistent with substantial stereochemical discrepancies between A2′p5′(c^3A)2′p5′A and the parent core (2′,5′) trimer whereas a specific recognition of N3 atom of mid-adenosine (A2) is unlikely. The extensive conformational analysis of c^3A-substituted core trimers compared to the initial parent core trimer showed close stereochemical resemblance between the parent core trimer and (c^3A)2′p5′A2′p5′A and A2′p5′A2′p5′(c^3A) analogs which is a strong evidence of syn orientation of the base with respect to the glycoside bond. Conversely, A2′p5′(c^3A)2′p5′A analog deviated rather significantly from the spatial arrangement of the parent core trimmer. The extensive conformational analysis of the c^3A-substituted core trimers versus the parent natural core trimer displayed close stereochemical similarity between the natural core trimer and (c^3A)2′p5′A2′p5′A and A2′p5′A2′p5′(c^3A) analogs, thereby strong evidences for the syn base orientation about the glycosyl bond of the c^3A residue of the latter were found. On the contrary, an analog A2′p5′(c^3A)2′p5′A displayed rather essential deviations from the spatial arrangement of the parent natural core trimer.

Synthesis data of 2-5A analogs containing 6-(benzylamino)purine riboside (AdoBn), a nucleoside with cytokinin activity are of interest. The second type of modification of the heterocyclic base was a replacement for virazole (ribavirin), a synthetic nucleoside that exhibits a wide range of antiviral activity against a wide variety of viruses. Compounds with high antiviral activity were found among the obtained oligomers. Studies of biological properties exhibited by these 2-5A analogs [23, 24] showed that these compounds had HIV-1 reverse transcriptase inhibitory and recombinant human ribonuclease L activity [25]. Specifically, trimers containing AdoBn at any positions of the oligonucleotide chain have been shown to impede the HIV-1-induced formation of syncytium by 1500 times (vs. three times for 2′,5′A_3 parent trimer). It is also in evidence that all virazole-containing trimers at a concentration of 300 μmol have been shown to inhibit HIV-1 reverse transcriptase by 99.5–99.7% (33% for parent trimer). The ability of AdoBn-containing compounds to inhibit this enzyme is based on the position of the modified nucleoside unit in the oligomer chain and is greatest for the trimer containing the above moiety in the 5′-terminal position. The ability of the studied 2′,5′-oligonucleotides to activate recombinant human ribonuclease L defined as the percentage of poly(U)-3′-[^{32}P]pCp hydrolysis in the presence of these compounds also depends on the structure of these oligoadenylates. Thus, the trimer containing a virazole moiety in the 5′-terminal position of the chain inhibited ribonuclease L by 87.7%

(50% for the parent trimer). AdoBn-containing compounds as the 5′-terminal and central link—by 37.4% and 34.8%, respectively, whereas the heterobase modified 2′-terminal unit of oligoadenylates resulted in a complete loss of ability to activate ribonuclease L [25].

3. (2′-5′)Oligoadenylates modified in the carbohydrate moiety

3.1 The role of structural and stereochemical factors in binding and activation of RNase L

The synthesis of parent 2-5A analogs modified in the carbohydrate moiety and the study of their physicochemical and biological properties helped to establish the role of structural and stereochemical factors of this unique class of cell biomolecules.

The substitution of ribose 3′-OH groups of ppp(A2′p5′)$_2$A with hydrogen proved that 3′-OH groups of (A2) moiety are essential for biological activity (**Figure 3**). However, this group is perhaps required for degradation by 2′-5′-phosphodiesterase since (A2′p5)$_2$A with (A2) substituted by xyloadenosine was resistant to 2′-5′-phosphodiesterase activity [26]. For 2′-5′-phosphodiesterase, 3′-OH groups of the second residue and free 2′- and 3′-OH groups of the 2′-terminal residue [27–30] are required.

The results of examinations to assess relationship between the structure and spatial arrangement (stereochemistry), on the one hand, and the biological properties of 2-5A analogs, on the other hand, clearly showed that the known properties can be enhanced or new properties can be added by changing the structure and/or stereochemistry of their molecules. For example, the use of fluorodeoxyadenylates, parent oligomer analogs, in which adenosine moieties are consecutively substituted by a conformationally rigid fluoronucleoside molecule for enzyme reaction tests allowed to differentiate the role of structural and stereochemical factors and demonstrate the effect of molecule stereochemistry on their biological properties [31].

Substitution of the 3′-hydroxyl group of adenosine furanose ring with a fluorine atom in two different configurations, *ribo* (A_F) and *xylo* (A^F), contributes to the overriding population of different conformations of the pentofuranose moiety due to stereochemical differences in the gauche effects of the fluorine atom and other electronegative substituents of furanose rings. It was demonstrated that the conformational features of individual fluoronucleosides A_F and A^F, which are mainly in the

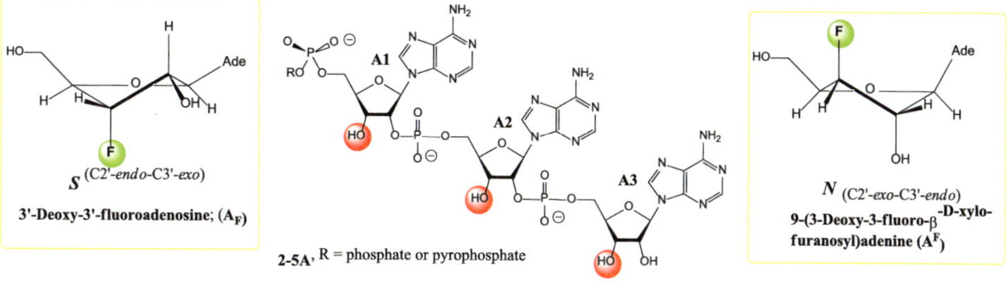

Figure 3.
Stereochemical structures of 3′-fluoro-ribo-adenosine (A_F), 3′-fluoro-xylo-adenosine (A^F), and the structure of 5′-phosphates of the 2′,5′-oligoadenylic acid trimer.

N- or S-conformation, respectively, are also preserved in the respective fluoronucleoside moiety of the trimer. These datademonstrated that the fluorine atom present in the carbohydrate part of the molecule is a key factor of the conformation of these molecules [31].

Stereochemical features of 2-5A *xylo*- and *ribo*-fluorodeoxy analogs make these compounds unique stereochemical analogs of the parent oligomer, which enables to discriminate the role of structural and stereochemical factors in biological processes. Indeed, on the one hand, a pair of A_F and A^F substituted analogs in a certain position of the chain is structurally related to 3′-deoxyadenosine (cordycepin) analogs, while on the other hand, the sugar rings A_F and A^F are in different conformations, S and N, respectively. These stereochemical differences between A_F and A^F are preserved when included in the (2′-5′) oligomer molecule instead of adenosine, and determine largely its stereochemistry. The *syn↔anti* orientation change of the heterocyclic base of A_F and A^F fluoronucleosides with prevalent syn- or anti-conformers, respectively, results in a variety of stacking interactions of heterocyclic bases and thereby changed oligonucleotide chain conformation as a whole. The introduction *of xylo*-fluoronucleoside (A^F) into the central (A2) 2-5A moiety produced an oligomer more resistant to (2′,5′)-phosphodiesterase compared to the parent trimer. At the same time, the presence of 3′-deoxy-, 3′-fluoro-*xylo*(A^F), or 3′-fluoro-*ribo*(A_F) adenosine in the (A3) moiety of oligoadenylate produced different degrees of hydrolysis despite their structural resemblance suggesting the role of the spatial arrangement of the molecule in the recognition thereof by phosphodiesterase active site [32].

The study of the ability of 2-5A fluorodeoxyanalogs to bind and activate RNase L showed that the analog whose fluorine atom in the *xylo*-configuration in the mid-moiety is nine times more active than the parent mediator, 2-5A and about 280 times more effective than isomeric *ribo*-trimer [32–34]. The results suggest that *anti↔syn* stereochemical differences between pppAA(A_F) and pppAA(A^F), on the one hand, and related 8-bromo- and -methyl-analogs, on the other hand, cause differences in the degree of RNase L activation. Data presented in [32–34] suggest the *syn*-orientation is a major contribution to this process. The pppA(A^F)A_F poor ability to activate RNase L supports this assumption.

It is noteworthy that 2-5A fluorine-substituted analogs are important for the analysis of stereochemical patterns of RNase L activation. The *syn*-orientation of the base both at 5′- terminal of the oligomer and in the central site and the prevalent *N*-conformation of pentofuranose residues are probably required to form a productive complex between the enzyme, mediator, and substrate. In addition, the *syn*-orientation of the base in (A3) moiety of the oligomer is positive for RNase L activation. These reasonably substantiated assumptions are quite paradoxical and a question suggests itself: could this unusual *syn*-orientation of bases being in the transient state during RNase L activation be the second - after the unusual (2′-5′) phosphodiester bond in the oligomer—unique property of this mediator?

The *syn*-orientation of the heterocyclic base in (A1) or (A2) units of the oligomer chain, together with the predominant *N*-conformation of pentofuranose residues, is obviously required to form a productive complex between the enzyme, mediator, and substrate. The *syn*-orientation of the base in (A3) moiety of the oligomer is also positive for RNase L activation. The trimer stereochemical features have been established to be pivotal in shaping RNase L binding and activation rather than the presence of C3′-OH group in 2-5A (A2) moiety.

3.2 Influence of structural (stereochemical) features of 3′-fluoroanalogs 2-5A on human NK cell lytic activity

The 2-5A system is not probably responsible for all interferon (INF) biological effects, however, varied evidence suggest that 2-5A, as well as 5′-dephosphorylated analogs are involved in various biochemical processes in animal cells including INF antiviral effect [35]. The INF ability to regulate lytic activity of parent killer cells (NK cells) [36, 37] is considered one of the key factors of INF antitumor effect [38]. It is noteworthy that NK cells are responsible for lysis of virtually any tumor and virally infected cells irrespective of antibodies or complement with no prior immunization needed [39, 40].

(2′-5′)Oligoadenylates, similarly to IFN, increase the NK cell lytic activity at an optimum concentration of 50 μM thus mimicking IFN action [41]. The study of effects produced by the parent trimer, A_3, and 3′-deoxyadenosine analog (3′dA_3) on NK cells showed that the increased NK cell activity is typical only for oligomers with a (2′-5′) phosphodiester bond. The (3′-5′)oligoadenylic acid trimer, (3′-5′)A_3 produced no effect on NK cell lytic activity even at a concentration of 300 μM. Adenosine and 3′-deoxyadenosine at a concentration of 150 μM also did not change NK cell activity, which rules out the effect of trimers as depot forms of nucleosides. It was assumed that the stereochemistry of (3′-5′)- and (2′-5′) phosphodiester bonds caused differences in the effects on NK cell lytic activity of these oligomers [41].

Based on these data, similar activity of A_3 and $(3'dA)_3$ in respect to NK cells seems unexpected. Indeed, both trimers are widely different in their spatial structure [31, 42]—the parent trimer being a conformationally flexible molecule, and for $(3'dA)_3$, only one spatial structure is predominantly occupied. Apparently, the $(3'dA)_3$ molecule is not more rigid thermodynamically compared to the parent trimer, A_3, and is capable of taking a spatial arrangement similar to that of the parent trimer when interacting with NK cells.

The effect of conformationally different molecules of *xylo* and *ribo* 3′-fluorodeoxyanalogs of (2′-5′)oligoadenylic acid on human parent killer (NK cells) was studied [43, 44]. Treatment of human effector NK cells with fluorodeoxyanalogs 2-5A has been generally shown to result in a significantly augmented cytotoxic activity toward target cells. Moreover, the degree of augmentation in NK cell activity varied significantly and depended on the conformation of the fluorodeoxyanalog (**Table 1**). Stereochemistry of (2′-5′)$(A^F)A_2$ and (2′-5′)$A(A^F)A$ trimers is determined by the predominant population of the furanose ring N-conformation and *syn*-orientation of the heterocyclic base around the glycosidic bond of A^F fragment. Relevant *ribo*-isomers, (2′-5′)$(A_F)A_2$ and (2′-5′)$A(A_F)A$ are similar to the parent trimer, (2′-5′)A_3, having *anti*-conformation of all heterobases yet rigid S-conformation of A_F furanose ring. All 2-5A *ribo*-fluorodeoxyanalogs were much more active on NK cells compared to *xylo*-analogs or the parent mediator, which is obviously due to a closer conformational resemblance of *ribo*- fluorodeoxyanalogs with the parent oligomer compared to isomeric *xylo*-analogs.

3.3 Effect of 2-5A fluorodeoxyanalogs on macrophage phagocytic activity

Another type of immune cells, mononuclear phagocytes (MPs) are cells, which are directly engaged in the formation of humoral and cellular immune responses. Their

(2′-5′) Oligoadenylate	LU_{20}*	Increased activity (%)**	LU_{30}*	Increased activity (%)**	LU_{50}*	Increased activity (%)**
Control	11.0	0	7.1	0	2.0	0
A_3	16.2	47	10.0	41	4.5	125
$(A^F)A_2$	8.0	−27	6.7	−5.6	2.0	0
$A(A^F)A$	10.0	−9	7.1	0	3.8	90
$A_2(A^F)$	16.0	46	9.4	32	4.2	108
$(A_F)A_2$	16.6	51	10.0	41	5.0	150
$A(A_F)A$	14.3	30	10.0	41	5.5	175
$A_2(A_F)$	11.5	4.5	8.3	17	4.5	125
$A(A^F)(A_F)$	12.2	11	8.0	13	4.3	115

**One lytic unit was assumed equal to the number of effector cell (natural killers) lysing 20% (LU_{20}), 30% (LU_{30}), and 50% (LU_{50}), respectively, of target cells during the study period. K-562 erythroleukemia cells were used as target cells and labeled with a non-radioactive chelate complex of europium diethylenetriaminepentaacetate (EuDTPA).*
***The percentage of increased lytic activity of N-lymphocytes was calculated by the formula: {[(LE/10^6 treated cells/ LE/10^6 control cells)] - 1} x 100.*

Table 1.
Effect of 3′-fluorodeoxyanalogs on NK-lymphocyte activity.

phagocytic activity entailing absorption and killing of certain types of microorganisms is one of many results of MP functioning.

The study of the effect of 2-5A on MPs showed that 2-5A analogs should have three phosphate residues at the 5′-end and at least three adenosine moieties to increase macrophage phagocytic activity. Moreover, it was found that MPs of various animal species have a 2-5A receptor, which has a high specificity. Substitution of adenosine moiety for inosine did not contribute to binding to the 2-5A receptor and thus did not increase macrophage phagocytic activity [45, 46].

Compound	Concentration 1×10^{-10} (M)		Compound	Concentration 1×10^{-6} (M)	
	I_{CL}(%)	relative activity		I_{CL}(%)	relative activity
$pppA_3$	46	1.0	A_3	31	1.0
$ppp(A^F)A_2$	56	1.2	$(A^F)A_2$	27	0.9
$pppA(A^F)A$	37	0.8	$A(A^F)A$	16	0.5
$pppA_2(A^F)$	34.5	0.75	$A_2(A^F)$	21	0.7
$ppp(A_F)A_2$	92	2.0	$(A_F)A_2$	40	1.3
$pppA(A_F)A$	57.5	1.25	$A(A_F)A$	43	1.4
$pppA_2(A_F)$	69	1.5	$A_2(A_F)$	42	1.35
$pppA(A^F)(A_F)$	31	0.67			

Values shown have been obtained from six to nine independent experiments. The phagocytic activity of macrophages was expressed in terms of the chemiluminescence index: $I_{CL}(\%) = \frac{CL_2 - CL_1}{CL_1} \cdot 100$, where CL_1 is the maximum chemiluminescence (mV) of native P388D1 cells and CL2 is the maximum chemiluminescence (mV) of activated P388D1 cells.

Table 2.
Effect of fluorodeoxyanalogs 2-5Aa on the phagocytic activity of mouse macrophages of the P388D1 line.

It was demonstrated that all 2-5A *ribo*-fluorodeoxyanalogs were much more superior in activating P388D1 cells than *xylo*-analogs, and the parent oligomer [47, 48]. Probably, *anti*-conformation of the heterocyclic base with the dominant S-conformation of carbohydrate moieties is more preferable for 2-5A receptor of P388D1 cells compared to the parent trimer where the furanose ring is located in the dynamic S↔N equilibrium with prevalent *anti*-orientation of adenine bases [31]. Conformational rigidity of the carbohydrate ring of the xylonucleoside, A^F, which was found to be largely occupied in *N*-conformation along with *syn*-orientation of the base resulted in reduced activation of P388D1 cells induced by (2′-5′) oligoadenylates. However, significant differences exist between *xylo*-and *ribo*-analogs in their ability to increase phagocytic activity (**Table 2**).

4. (2′-5′)oligoadenylates containing *epoxy*-groups rather than 2′,3′-cis-diol group

The use of 2-5A analogs in kidney transplant surgeries in monkeys was demonstrated in [49]. Based on the results, 2-5A analogs were selected from a variety of synthesized compounds in which 2′(3′)-terminal adenosine moiety of the molecule was substituted with 9-(2,3-anhydro-β-D-ribofuranosyl)adenine [(2′,5′)A_2A_{RA}] or 9-(2,3-anhydro-β-D-lyxofuranosyl)adenine [(2′,5′)A_2 A^{LA}] (**Figure 4**).

These compounds (*i*) were more resistant to snake venom phosphodiesterase compared to the parent trimer, (2′,5′)A_3, ($t_{1/2}$ hydrolysis 16 h, 10.5 h, and 27 min, respectively), *(ii)* exhibited no toxicity in mice at a concentration of 1 mg per kg of body weight and *(iii)* showed peculiar characteristics of lymphocytes in blastogenic response in the presence of mitogens during the *in vitro* experiments (**Tables 3** and **4**). The effects produced by these isomeric analogs were much more pronounced and they differed from 2′-5′A_3 in their response to concanavalin A (Con A)- and lipopolysaccharide (LPS)-induced lymphocyte blastogenic response (**Table 3**). Con A primarily stimulates T-lymphocyte division whereas LPS acts on β-lymphocytes.

Biochemical test results convincingly demonstrated the potential of two analogs (2′,5′)A_3, (2′,5′)$A_2A_{RA,}$ and (2′,5′)A_2A^{LA} for the treatment of various conditions including those associated with T-cell immunodeficiency diseases, autoimmune diseases, viral infections, lymphocytic malignant transformations, graft failure prevention following the bone marrow transplantation and perhaps, complications associated with the recipient's transplant rejection.

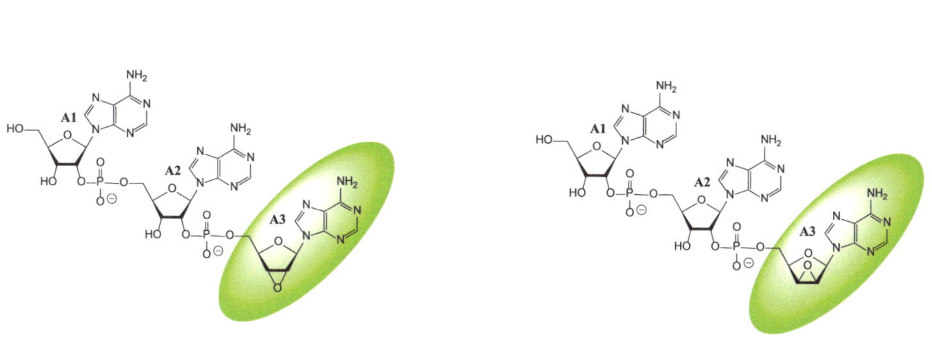

(2',5')A_2A_{RA} (2',5') A_2A^{LA}

Figure 4.
2-5A dephosphorylated analogs containing epoxy-groups rather than 2′,3′-cis-diol group in A3 moiety in ribo-[(2′,5′)A_2A_{RA}] and lyxo-(2′,5′)A_2A^{LA}] configurations.

Mitogen	DNA synthesis by incorporation of [^{3}H]-thymidine (pulse/min)			
	Control	Connection (5×10^{-6} M)		
		$(2',5')A_3$	$(2',5')A_2A_{RA}$	$(2',5')$ A_2A^{LA}
Con A (5 µg/mL)	22.296	18.934	16.399	15.749
LPS (0.1 µg/mL)	27.133	1.588	21.464	10.828

Table 3.
Comparative analysis of in vitro mammalian lymphocyte blastogenic response.

Control	DNA synthesis by incorporation of [^{3}H]-thymidine (pulse/min)				
	Concentration $(2',5')A_2A_{RA}$ (M)*				
	5×10^{-6}	5×10^{-7}	5×10^{-8}	5×10^{-9}	5×10^{-10}
Con A (5 µg/mL) 5.428 *[5.108]*	1.733 *[7732]*	3.865 *[2237]*	5.383 *[1355]*	1.599 *[6915]*	777 *[1425]*
LPS (0.1 µg/mL) 10.766 *[5.513]*	7.665 *[131]*	6.018 *[292]*	4.767 *[655]*	7.348 *[3342]*	672 *[1213]*

Data for $(2',5')A_3$ at the same concentration are shown in square brackets.

Table 4.
Concentration dependence of in vitro lymphocyte blastogenic response as affected by $(2',5')A_2A_{RA}$ vs. $(2',5')A_3$.

The potential use of $(2',5')A_2A_{RA}$ and $(2',5')A_2A^{LA}$ analogs for kidney transplantation in rabbits and monkeys has been thoroughly studied [49]. Daily intravenous injection of $(2',5')$ A_2A_{RA} to rabbits at a dose of 5 µg/kg of body weight ensures the normal functioning of the transplanted kidney in 4 out of 10 animals within 3 months. The lymphocyte blastogenic response in positive rabbits was suppressed by about 10 times by concanavalin (Con A) stimulation within 2 weeks after surgery.

Immunotropic activity of $(2',5')A_2A_{RA}$ and $(2',5')A_2A^{LA}$ analogs vs. $(2',5')A_3$ was assessed in a group of monkeys aged 4. The parent trimer $(2',5')A_3$ showed no immunosuppressive activity at a concentration of 0.5 mg/kg (data not shown). Moreover, a single intravenous injection resulted in a ~ 50% increase in T-helpers and T-killers responsible for the transplant rejection.

The results of the $(2',5')A_2A_{RA}$ study are summarized in **Table 5**. It should be emphasized that the analog inhibits interleukin-2 (IL-2) and T-lymphocyte subpopulation and concurrently stimulates αIFN and γIFN in blood lymphocytes for 2–3 weeks with a single injection at a concentration of 50 µg/kg (**Table 5**) and 25 µg/kg (data not shown).

After cross-allotransplantation of the kidney in two groups of monkeys, they were followed up for 3 months. Of note, normal functioning of the transplanted kidney occurred within 10 hours after the operation.

The data shown in **Table 5** suggest selective suppression of T-lymphocyte subpopulation immediately after surgery, subsequent recovery to preoperative levels followed by mild reduction of T-helper and T-killer populations, and slight increase in T-suppressor count. This trend persisted throughout the postoperative follow-up period.

Experiments in monkeys have shown that intravenous $(2'-5')A_2A_{RA}$ given every 48 hours at a concentration of 50 µg/kg provides immunosuppression, protects the

Type of assay	Days after the introduction of the trimmer					
	0	1	2	8	12	21
IgG (g/L)	9.6	7.8	15.0	14.8		13.2
IgA (g/L)	2.8	2.7	0.8	0.9		0.4
IgM (g/L)	0.6	0.5	1.1	0.9		0.8
T-helpers (%)	30	29	15	5.0	7.0	30.6
T-suppressors (%)	43	31	19	7.4	13	44
T-killers (%)	12	9	7	4.4	9	19.3
αIFN*) (plasma)	16	32	4	—	4	4
γIFN*) (lymphocytes)	4	8	32	—	32	8
αIFN*) (lymphocytes)	32	32	64	—	64	32
IL- 2	8	4	4	—	4	4

Units of IFN per 10.000 lymphocytes.

Table 5.
Effect of a single intravenous injection of trimer (2′,5′)A_2A_{RA} at a dose of 50 μg/kg on the immune system of macaque Rh monkeys.

Type of assay	2 days pre-oper. 50 μg/kg	Days postoperation				
		1	5	8	13	18
IgG (g/L)	13	—	12.2	12.8	—	—
IgA (g/L)	0.4	—	2.1	2.5	—	—
IgM (g/L)	0.8	—	0.8	0.9	—	—
T-helpers (%)	30	8	39.9	32	34.7	14.5
T-suppressors (%)	44	40.6	44	47	47.7	57.5
T-killers (%)	19	5	19	22	22.6	16

Table 6.
Effect of intravenous administrations of (2′-5′)A_2A_{RA} (50 μg/kg) on the immune system of macaque Rh. Monkeys after kidney transplantation. Intravenous administration (50 μg/kg) on day 2, 6, and 12 after surgery and every sixth day thereafter.

graft from rejection, and resumes normal functioning of the kidney transplant. T-helper and T-killer counts during the first two most critical postoperative weeks were reduced by 2–3 times remaining at 30% of a normal value (**Table 6**).

5. Conclusions

As a result of studies to clarify the relationship between the structure and spatial organization (stereochemistry), on the one hand, and the biological properties of analogs 2-5A, on the other one, it was convincingly shown that by changing the structure and/or stereochemistry of their molecules, it is possible to achieve either strengthening of known or giving new properties. The different functional groups of each individual 2-5A nucleotide fragment make a highly specific contribution to the binding and activation of RNase L, as well as to hydrolytic stability.

The use of conformationally rigid 3′-fluorodeoxyanalogs 2-5A and core trimer 2-5A on the example of human NK lymphocytes and mouse macrophages of the $P388D_1$ line allows us to evaluate the influence of structural and stereochemical factors on the cells of the immune system. *Ribo*-fluorodeoxyanalogs 2-5A had a more significant activating effect on human NK lymphocytes and phagocytic activity than *xylo*-analogs or a natural mediator, which is probably due to the closer conformational similarity of *ribo*-fluorodeoxyanalogs with a natural oligomer than with isomeric *xylo*-analogs.

Analogs 2-5A, $(2',5')A_2A_{RA}$, and $(2',5')A_2A^{LA}$ are undoubtedly of considerable interest for transplantology as drugs that prevent kidney rejection, ensure the normal functioning of the transplanted kidney and at the same time do not increase the level of T-helper and T-killer cells in experimental animals in postoperative period.

Undoubtedly, the search for approaches to the directed regulation of the natural protective function of the body with the help of analogs of the core trimer 2-5A can lead to the detection of compounds with high therapeutic potential.

Author details

Elena Kalinichenko
Institute of Bioorganic Chemistry of National Academy of Sciences of Belarus, Minsk, Belarus

*Address all correspondence to: kalinichenko@iboch.by

References

[1] Williams BRG, Kerr IM. Inhibition of protein synthesis by 2′-5′ linked adenine oligonucleotides in intact cells. Nature. 1978;**276**:88-90. DOI: 10.1038/276088a0

[2] Malathi K, Dong B, Gale M, Silverman RH. Small self-RNA generated by RNase L amplifies antiviral innate immunity. Nature. 2007;**448**:816-819

[3] Cooper DA, Banerjee S, Chakrabarti A, Garcia-Sastre A, Hesselberth JR, Silverman RH, et al. RNase L targets distinct sites in influenza a virus RNAs. Journal of Virology. 2015;**89**:764-776

[4] Ezelle HJ, Malathi K, Hassel BA. The roles of RNase-L in antimicrobial immunity and the cytoskeleton-associated innate response. International Journal of Molecular Sciences. 2016;**17**:74. DOI: 10.3390/ijms17010074

[5] Drappier M, Michiels T. Inhibition of the OAS/RNase L pathway by viruses. Current Opinion in Virology. 2015;**15**:19-26

[6] Kwon Y-C et al. The ribonuclease L-dependent antiviral roles of human 2′,5′-oligoadenylate synthetase family members against hepatitis C virus. FEBS Letters. 2013;**587**(2):156-164. DOI: 10.1016/j.febslet.2012.11.010

[7] Ghosh A, Shao L, Sampath P, Zhao B, Patel NV, Zhu J, et al. Oligoadenylate-synthetase-family protein OASL inhibits activity of the DNA sensor GAS during DNA virus infection to limit interferon production. Immunity. 2019;**50**(1):51-63

[8] Drappier M et al. A novel mechanism of RNase L inhibition: Theiler's virus L* protein prevents 2-5A from binding to RNase L. PLoS Pathogens. 2018;**14**(4):e1006989

[9] Rusch L, Zhou A, Silverman RH. Mint: Caspase-dependent apoptosis by 2′,5′-oligoadenylate activation of RNase L is enhanced by IFN-b. Journal of Interferon & Cytokine Research. 2000;**20**:1091-1100

[10] Manivannan P, Reddy V, Mukherjee S. RNase L Induces Expression of A Novel Serine/Threonine Caspase-dependent apoptosis by 2′,5′-oligoadenylate activation of RNase L is enhanced by IFN-b. International Journal of Molecular Research. 2019;**20**:3535

[11] Lengyel P. Biochemistry of interferons and their actions. Annual Review of Biochemistry. 1982;**51**:251-282. DOI: 10.1146/annurev.bi.51.070182.001343

[12] Wood ER, Bledsoe R, Chai J, Daka P, Deng H, Ding Y, et al. The role of phosphodiesterase 12 (PDE12) as a negative regulator of the innate immune response and the discovery of antiviral inhibitors. The Journal of Biological Chemistry. 2015;**290**:19681-19696

[13] Torrence PF, Imai J, Jamoulle J-C, Lesiak K. Biological activity of molecular dissections and transformations of 2-5A. Chemical Script. 1986;**26**:191-197

[14] Imai J, Lesiak K, Torrence PF. Respective roles of each of the purine N-6 amino groups of 5′-O-triphosphoryladenylyl(2′-5′)adenylyl(2′-5′)adenosine in binding to and activation of RNase L. Journal of Biological Chemistry. 1985;**260**:1390-1393

[15] Torrence P.F, Imai J, Lesiak K, Jamoulle J.-C, Sawai H. Oligonucleotide structural parameters that influence binding of 5′-O-triphosphoadenyl-(2′–5′)

adenyl(2′–5′)adenosine to the 5′-O-triphosphoadenyl-(2′–5′) adenyl(2′–5′)-adenosine-dependent endoribonuclease: Chain length, phosphorylation state and heterocyclic base. Journal of Medicinal Chemistry 1984;**27**:726-733. DOI: 10.1021/jm00372a004

[16] Kitade Y, Alster DK, Pabuccuoglu A, Torrence PF. Uridine analogs of 2′,5′-oligoadenylates: On the biological role of the middle base of 2-5A trimer. Bioorganic Chemistry. 1991;**19**:283-299. DOI: 10.1016/0045-2068(91)90054-s

[17] Van den Hoogen Y, Th HCM, Brozda D, Lesiak K, Torrence PE, Altona C. Conformational analysis of brominated pA2′-5′A2′-5′a analogs. An NMR and model-building study. European Journal of Biochemistry. 1989;**182**:629-637. DOI: 10.1016/0045-2068(91)90054-S

[18] Kitade Y, Nakata Y, Hirota K, Maki Y, Pabuccuoglu A, Torrence P.F. 8-Methyladenosine-substitutedanalogues of 2-5A: Synthesis and their biological activities. Nucleic Acids Research 1991; 19: 4103-4108. doi:10.1093/nar/19.15.4103

[19] Kanou M, Ohomori H, Takaku H, Yokoyama S, Kawai G. Chemical synthesis and biological activities of analogues of 2′,5′-oligoadenylates containing 8-substituted adenosine derivatives. Nuicleic Acids Res. 1990;**18**:4439-3446. DOI: 10.1093/nar/18.15.4439

[20] Mikhailopulo I.A, Kalinichenko E.N, Podkopaeva T.L, Rosemeyer H, Seela F. Synthesis of 1-deazaadenosine analogues of (2′→5′)ApApA. Nucleosides & Nucleotides 1996;**15**(1-3):445-464. DOI: 10.1080/07328319608002397

[21] Player MR, Kalinichenko EN, Podkopaeva TL, Mikhailopulo IA, Seela F, Torrence PF. Dissection of the roles of adenine ring nitrogen (N-1) and exocyclic amino (N-6) moieties in the interaction of 2-5A with RNase L. Biochemical and Biophysical Research Communications. 1998;**245**(2):430-434. DOI: 10.1006/bbrc.1998.8451

[22] Kalinichenko EN, Podkopaeva TL, Budko EV, Seela F, Dong B, Silverman R, et al. 3-Deazaadenosine analogues of p5′A2′p5′A2′p5′A: Synthesis, stereochemistry, and the roles of adenine ring Nitrogen-3 in the interaction with RNase L. Bioorganic & Medicinal Chemistry. 2004;**12**:3637-3647. DOI: 10.1016/j.bmc.2004.04.021

[23] Kvasyuk EI, Kulak TI, Mikhailopulo IA, Suhadolnik RJ, Henderson EE, Horvath SE, et al. Synthesis and biological activity of new 2′,5′-oligonucleotides. Nucleosides & Nucleotides. 1997;**16**(7-9):1351-1354. DOI: 10.1080/07328319708006186

[24] Kvasyuk EI, Kulak TI, Zinchenko AI, Barai VN, Mikhailopulo IA. 6-Benzyladenosine analogues of (A2′p)2A: Synthesis and activity against tobacko mosaik virus. Russian Journal of Bioorganic Chemistry. 1996;**22**(3):208-214

[25] Kvasyuk EI, Kulak TI, Tkachenko OV, Sentyureva SL, Mikhaylopulo IA, Zinchenko AI, et al. Proceedings of the Academy of Sciences of the BSSR. Series in Chemical Science. 1996;**3**:73-79

[26] Kvasyuk EI, Kulak TI, Tkachenko OV, Sentyureva SL, Mikhailopulo IA, Suhadolnik RJ, et al. Synthesis and biological activity of New Base-modified (2′-5′)Oligoadenylate trimers. Helvetica Chimica Acta. 1997;**80**:1053-1060. DOI: 10.1002/hlca.19970800404

[27] Torrence PF, Alster D, Huss S, Gosselin G. Degradation by the 2′,5′-phosphodiesterase activity of

mouse cells requires the presence of a ribo hydroxyl group in the penultimate position of the oligonucleotide substrate. FEBS Letters. 1987;**212**:267-270. DOI: 10.1016/0014-5793(87)81358-3

[28] Johnston MI, Hearl WG. Purification and characterization of a 2′-phosphodiesterase from bovine spleen. Journal of Biological Chemistry. 1987;**262**:8377-8382

[29] Bayard B, Bisbal C, Silhol M, Cnockaert J, Huez G, Lebleu B. Increased stability and antiviral activity of 2′-O-phosphoglyceryl derivatives of (2′-5′)oligo(adenylate). European Journal of Biochern. 1984;**142**:291-298. DOI: 10.1111/j.1432-1033.1984.tb08284.x

[30] Baglioni C et al. Analogs of (2′-5′) oligo(A). Endonuclease activation and inhibition of protein synthesis in intact cells. The Journal of Biological Chemistry. 1981;**256**:3253-3257

[31] Van den Boogaart JE, Kalinichenko EN, Podkopaeva TL, Mikhailopulo IA, Altona C. Conformational analysis of 3′-fluorinated A2′-5′A2′-5′a fragments. Relation between conformation and biological activity. European Journal of Biochemistry. 1994;**221**:759-768

[32] Kalinichenko EN, Podkopaeva TL, Kelve M, Saarma M, Mikhailopulo IA. 3′-Fluoro-3′-deoxy analogs of 2-5A 5′-monophosphate: Binding to 2-5A-dependent endoribonuclease and susceptibility to (2′-5′)phosphodiesterase degradation. Biochemical Biophysical Research Communication. 1990;**167**:20-26

[33] Kalinichenko EN, Kelve M, Podkopaeva TL, Saarma M, Mikhailopulo IA. The study of the structural requirement for Rnase L activation by 3′-fluoro-3′-deoxy analogs of 2-5A. Journal of Interferon Research. 1993;**13**:88

[34] Kalinichenko EN, Podkopaeva TL, Poopeiko NE, Kelve M, Saarma M, Mikhailopulo IA, et al. Role of the stereochemistry of 3′-fluoro-3′-deoxy analogues of 2-5A in binding to and activation of the RNase L of mouse cells. Recueil Trav. Chim. Pays-Bas. 1995;**114**:43-50. DOI: 10.1002/recl.19951140202

[35] Charubala R, Pfleiderer W. Progress in Molecular and Subcellular Biology. Berlin; Heidelberg: Springer Verlag; 1994. pp. 114-138

[36] Lee SH, Kelley S, Stebbing N. Stimulation of natural killer cell activity and inhibition of proliferation of various leukemic cells by purified human leukocyte interferon subtypes. Cancer Research. 1982;**42**(4):1312-1316

[37] Herberman RB, Ortaldo JR, Timonen T. Assay of augmentation of natural killer cell activity and antibody-dependent cell-mediated cytotoxicity by interferon. Methods in Enzymology. 1981;**79**:477-484. DOI: 10.1007/BF00922756

[38] Reid LM, Minato N, Grosser I, Holland J, Kadish A, Bloom BR. Influence of anti-mouse interferon serum on the growth and metastasis of tumor cells persistently injected with virus and of human prostatic tumors in athymic nude mice. Proceedings of the National Academy Science USA. 1981;**78**(2):1171-1175. DOI: 10.1073/pnas.78.2.1171

[39] Whiteside TL, Herberman RB, Review SA. The role of natural killer cells in human disease. Clinical Immunology and Immunopathology. 1989;**53**:1-23. DOI: 10.1016/0090-1229(89)90096-2

[40] Herberman RB, Ortaldo JR. Natural killer cells: Their role in defenses against

disease. Science. 1981;**4516**:24-30. DOI: 10.1126/science.7025208

[41] Black PL, Henderson EE, Pfleiderer W, Charubala R, Suhadolnik RJ. 2′-5′-oligoadenylate trimer core and the cordycepin analog augment the tumorocidal activity of human natural killer cells. Journal of Immunology. 1984;**135**(5):2733-2777

[42] Doornbos J, Charubala R, Pfleiderer W, Altona C. Conformational analysis of the trinucleoside diphosphate 3′d(A2′-5′A2′-5′A). An NMR and CD study. Nucleic Acids Research. 1983;**11**(13):4569-4582

[43] Kelve M, Kalinichenko EN, Podkopaeva TL, Saarma M. 3′-Fluoro-3′-deoxy analogs of 2-5A trimer core: Influence on the lytic activity of human natural killer cells. Journal of Interferon Research. 1992;**12**(1):120

[44] Kalinichenko EN, Podkopaeva TL, Kelve M, Saarma M, Mikhailopulo IA. 3'-Deoxy-3′-fluoro analogs of core trimers of 2-5A: Effect on lytic activity of human NK-lymphocytes. Bioorganicheskaia Khimiia. 1999;**25**(4):282-289

[45] Bollang L, Liu X. Mechanism of interferon action. The discovery of pppA2p5A2p5A receptor. Scientia Sinica. 1985;**XXVIII**(7):697-706

[46] Bollang L, Liu X. Mechanism of interferon action. Structural requirement of ligand and cellular specificity of pppA2p5A2p5A receptor. Scientia Sinica. 1985;**XXVIII**(8):844-853

[47] Kalinichenko EN. Influence of 3′-deoxy-3′-fluorine trimer (2′-5′) oligoadenylic acid on the phagocytic activity of macrophages: Stereochemical aspect. Presiding NAS of Belarus. Ser. chem. 2000;**1**:79-84

[48] Kelve M, Kuusksalu A, Kalinichenko E. 3′-Fluoro-3′-deoxy analogs of 2-5A trimer: enhangement of the phagocytic activity of macrophages. In: 5 th International Congress on Cell Biology, Madrid (Spain) 26th-31st July, 1992. Madrid (Spain); 1992. p. 13

[49] Mikhailopulo IA, Tkachuk ZY, Baran EA, Tkachuk LV, Kozlov AV, Slukvin II, Kvasyuk EI et al. Synthesis and use of (2′,5′)oligoadenylate trimers modified at the 2′-terminus in kidney transplantation in rabbits and monkeys Nucleosides & Nucleotides. 1995;**14**(3-5):1105-1108

Section 2

New Generation of Oligonucleotide Technology

Chapter 4

Combinatorial Oligonucleotide FISH (COMBO-FISH): Computer Designed Probe Sets for Microscopy Research of Chromatin in Cell Nuclei

Michael Hausmann and Eberhard Schmitt

Abstract

Genome sequence databases of many species have been completed so that it is possible to apply an established technique of FISH (Fluorescence In Situ Hybridization) called COMBO-FISH (COMBinatorial Oligonucleotide FISH). It makes use of bioinformatic sequence database search for probe design. Oligonucleotides of typical lengths of 15–30 nucleotides are selected in such a way that they only co-localize at the given genome target. Typical probe sets of 20–40 stretches label about 50–250 kb specifically. The probes are either solely composed of purines or pyrimidines, respectively, for Hoogsteen-type binding, or of purines and pyrimidines together for Watson-Crick type binding. We present probe sets for tumor cell analysis. With an improved sequence database analysis and sequence search according to uniqueness, a novel family of probes repetitively binding to characteristic genome features like SINEs (Short Interspersed Nuclear Elements, e.g., ALU elements), LINEs (Long Interspersed Nuclear Elements, e.g., L1), or centromeres has been developed. All types of probes can be synthesized commercially as DNA or PNA probes, labelled by dye molecules, and specifically attached to the targets for microscopy research. With appropriate dyes labelled, cell nuclei can be subjected to super-resolution localization microscopy.

Keywords: DNA database analysis, computer designed oligonucleotide probes, specific fluorescence labeling of genome targets, fluorescence microscopy of chromosomes and cell nuclei, super-resolution localization microscopy for chromatin architecture research

1. Introduction

Although first models assuming that chromatin in the interphase nucleus is well organized in distinct territories and domains, can be found in the late 19th and early 20th centuries [1, 2], experimental methods of visualization of genome architecture were missing until the 1970s/1980s [3]. With the breakthrough of three-dimensional (3D) light microscopy, especially 3D fluorescence confocal laser scanning microscopy also developments of specific labeling techniques like fluorescence in situ hybridization (FISH; for review see [4]) started their story of success in genome research and medical diagnostics.

FISH is based on the principle that a DNA probe either amplified in bacteria or by PCR represents the nucleic acid sequence of a given target DNA in the cell nucleus or of a metaphase chromosome [5]. Such a probe has to be thermally or chemically denatured into single DNA strands (if not synthesized by PCR) that can bind complementary to the single, that is, denatured DNA strands of given targets [6, 7]. The probes are labeled with fluorochromes. If these single-stranded probe molecules are added in excess to the denatured target strands, they specifically bind to their complementary target DNA so that a DNA–DNA hybrid with fluorescence labeling is formed [8]. Using various probes labeled with fluorochromes of different colors, multi-target visualization can be processed simultaneously [5].

With automated methods for artificial synthesis of high-purity DNA or PNA [9] oligonucleotides, probe sets of custom-made oligonucleotides have become available for many genomic target sites. Also, highly repetitive sequences in centromeres or telomeres were labeled [10]. By means of so-called "oligopaint" probes (fluorescently-labeled single-stranded DNA oligonucleotides) covering target sites by huge amounts of oligonucleotides, sequential, highly specific labeling of various targets from 5 kb up to a few Mb was performed. Oligopaint procedures depend on molecular biology techniques while COMBO-FISH probe design is fully based on computer database investigations. Further details of oligopaint can be found in References [11–14].

Standard FISH probes as well as oligopainting probes work on probe-target base-pairing according to the Watson–Crick binding scheme, that is, the single-stranded probe complementarily binds to one target strand. This requires heat or chemical denaturation of the complete DNA in a cell nucleus [6, 7] which could impact the preservation of chromosome morphology and especially chromatin nano-structure [15]. In addition, FISH under vital conditions appears to be nearly impossible.

PNA oligonucleotide probes show a higher target affinity than DNA probes. This allows PNA probes sufficient access to DNA targets without additional heat denaturation, because native chromatin acts in an equilibrium state of single- and double-strand conformation [16]. Experimentally, this was only shown for repetitive DNA targets [17] but not in oligopainting experiments of complex targets.

In principle, COMBinatorial Oligonucleotide FISH (COMBO-FISH) potentially has several advantages over standard FISH and could also overcome all such drawbacks mentioned above. COMBO-FISH has been invented in the late 1990s [18] and experimentally realized in the early 2000s [19]. It only uses a few short oligonucleotides for specific labeling of a target. These COMBO-FISH probes can be synthesized as DNA or PNA sequences binding complementarily either as a Watson–Crick double-strand or as a Hoogsteen triple-strand [20–22] (**Figure 1**). A low number of probes labeling a target strand reduces synthesis costs and (triple)-strand binding without a strong denaturation step conserves chromatin morphology and organization with the nowadays advantage that the native chromatin structure can be analyzed on the nano-scale by super-resolution localization microscopy in 3D conserved cell nuclei [23–25].

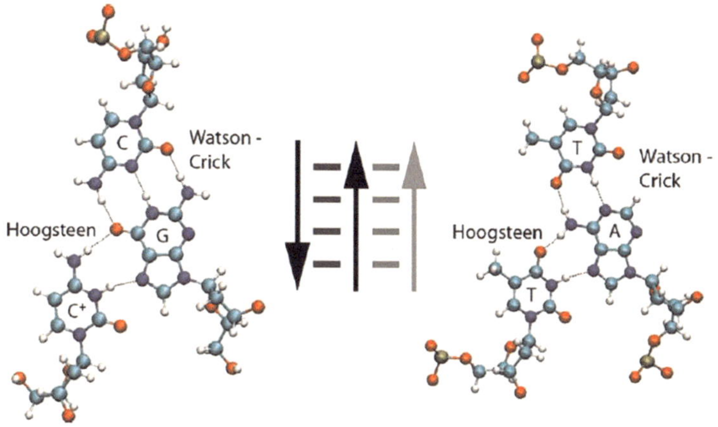

Figure 1.
*Snapshot of a molecular dynamics simulation showing Watson–Crick double-strand pairing and triplex structures of the two classical Hoogsteen pairs for parallel binding: C + *GC (left) and T*AT (right). Note: This figure was originally published in [20] and is reproduced with general permission of the publisher.*

2. COMBO-FISH: principle and applications

In contrast to standard FISH where probes are usually cut and amplified by molecular biology techniques, COMBinatorial Oligonucleotide FISH (COMBO-FISH) follows a completely different strategy for probe design [19, 20, 26, 27]. If a genome of a species is sequenced and the sequence is cataloged in a database, oligonucleotide probes can be searched and a set of probes can be designed in silico. Also, their specificity is controlled by computer analysis searching for all possible binding sites of each probe [20, 28, 29].

Any given genome target that should be specifically labeled, can be selected in a DNA sequence database and the numbers of the beginning and end nucleotides are determined exactly. This cannot only be done for human but also for any other species with completely known DNA sequences that can be read in established DNA database archives like NCBI.

The process works as follows [20]: firstly, the beginning and end numbers of a given target (for instance, a gene) are selected. Then oligonucleotide stretches of 15–30 distinct bases are determined in such a way that just the combination of those stretches is singularly co-localizing at the given target site. All binding sites of each probe are determined. Finally, several probe combinations may be excluded from consideration: (a) these are those that have accessory binding sites at other locations in a genome than at the given target site or (b) those that co-localize at several loci in the same genome (**Table 1**). In addition to these principles governing the basic probe selection, further characteristic features (experimental and theoretical) can be taken into account to ensure a stable homogenous hybridization protocol. Among these, the most important ones are oligonucleotide length, binding energy [28], homo-purine/-homo-pyrimidine sequences [30, 31], melting temperature [32], CG-content [32], etc. (see **Table 2** as an example). Typically, such oligonucleotide stretches included in a probe set have a length of 15–30 nucleotides each.

Several probe sets created according to this procedure (e.g., ABL, BCR, Her2neu, GRB7, AMACR, etc., see below) have been published or will be shown in the next chapter.

Gene	Position on chromosome	Base position	B	R
NRAS	1p13.2	4773158.4824158	62	35
AKT3	1q44	1714365.2069716	55	37
MSH2	2p22.3-p22.1	5331083.5503008	80	49
GNLY	2p12-q11	17,295,832..17300298	113	33
RASSF1	3p21.3	587,156..598306	134	61
FHIT	3p14.2	3106362.3371407	84	50
PIM1	6p21.2	27,935,054..27940329	101	52
ABCB1 (MDR)	7q21.1	12,367,353..12576743	85	54
MET	7q31	41,489,038..41613011	90	26
CMYC	8q24.12-q24.1	191,836..197827	113	57
CDKN2A(p16)	9p21	21,935,774..21963322	101	53
PTEN	10q23.3	897,571..1000507	66	41
ATM	11q22.3	11,636,339..11779887	44	27
KRAS2	12p11.2	2,778,774..2824914	69	43
RB1	13q14	17452380.17630614	64	34
PNN	14q13	19,564,443..19572199	52	32
SNRPNup	15q12	3595436.3750373	40	21
IGF1R	15q25-q26	297,646..606403	101	59
FANCA	16q24.3	610,999..690100	49	32
D17S125	17p12-p11.2	7,147,833..7148031	105	30
ERBB2	17	1593840.1622888	159	77
LAMA3	18q11.2	2,933,849..3024059	120	59
AKT2	19q13.l-q13.2	13,007,022..13060073	81	43
MYBL2	20q13.1	7,348,623..7398038	77	39
PTPN1	20q13.1-q13.2	14,179,798..14253995	78	45
ZNF217	20q13.2-q13.3	17236471.17252494	69	39
PCNT2	21qtel	3053753.3175376	71	38
PDGFB (SIS)	22q13.1	18,834,148..18855844	114	60
TBX1	22q11.2	2892106.2918996	64	38

Note: This table was originally published in [20] and is reproduced with general permission of the publisher.

Table 1.
Examples of COMBO-FISH target sites ("Gene"), their positions according to the banding annotation ("Positions on chromosome"), start and end position in the human data base ("Base position"), possible number of probes ("B") and the finally remaining specifically co-localizing probes ("R").

Finally, the computer-optimized probe set can be synthesized as DNA probes, PNA probes, SMART probes, or TINA (Twisted Intercalating Nuclear Acid) probes with high purity [30, 33–35]. PNA probes have a peptide backbone instead of a sugar–phosphate backbone of DNA. SMART probes also called molecular beacons consist of a stem-loop conformation quenching fluorescence by the closed loop until loop

Probe ID	Length (bp)	GC content (%)	Tm[a] (°C)	Molar mass (g/mol)	Sequence
AMACR1	**16**	**43.S**	**40.6**	**6110.2**	**AGG AAG AAG GGG AAA A**
AMACR2	16	43.8	34.4	6110.2	GGA GGA AAA GAG AAA G
AMACR7	15	40.0	31.2	5781.0	AGA AAG AAA AGA GGG
AMACR9	17	35.3	30.6	6068.1	CTT CTC TTC TTT CTC TT
AMACR10	17	58.8	45.3	6471.5	GAA GAG GAA AGG GAG GG
AMACR11	16	37.5	37.9	5763.9	TCT TCC TTT TCC CTT T
AMACR12	16	43.8	30.6	6110.2	GGA GAG AAG AAA GAA G
AMACR13	17	76.5	57.9	6519.5	GGG GGG AAG GGG AGG GA
AMACR14	15	66.7	43.3	5399.7	CCC CTC CCT CTT TCC
AMACR16	16	62.5	45.5	5703.9	TTC CTC CCT CCC CTC T
AMACR17	15	40.0	31.7	5459.7	TTT CTC CTC TTT TCC
AMACR23	15	60.0	37.0	5829.0	GAG AAG AAG AGG GGG
AMACR26	15	53.3	37.0	5813.0	AAG GAA GGA AGA GGG
AMACR27	15	53.3	29.9	5813.0	GAA GAG AAG GGA GAG
AMACR28	16	37.5	34.6	6094.2	AGG GAA AGA AGA AAA G
AMACR30	15	66.7	39.9	5845.0	GAA GAG GGG GGA GAG
AMACR31	15	53.3	34.0	5429.7	CCT CCT TTC CTT CTC
AMACR32	15	50.0	32.9	5733.9	CTC CTC TTT CTC CTC T
AMACR33	15	33.3	28.2	5765.0	AAA AGA AGG AAA GAG
AMACR36	16	43.8	37.3	5748.9	TCC CTT TTC TTC TCC T
AMACR37	17	41.2	34.1	6053.1	CTT TCC TCT TCT TTC TC
AMACR38	17	41.2	36.9	6423.5	AGA GAA AGA GGA AAA GG
AMACR39	17	52.9	42.2	6455.5	AGA GGA AGA AAG GGA GG
AMACR40	16	37.5	34.6	5763.9	CTT CTT CCT TCC TTT T
AMACR43	15	46.7	34.0	5797.0	AGA GGA GAA AGG GAA
AMACR45	15	40.0	27.1	5459.7	CTC TCT CCT TCT TTT
AMACR46	17	52.9	42.3	6023.1	TTT CTC CTC CCC TCT CT
AMACR48	15	46.7	34.7	5444.7	TCT TCT TCC TTT CCC
AMACR50	15	40.0	34.9	5781.0	AAA AGG GAG GAA AAG

Note: This table was originally published under CC BY license in [32].
[a]Melting temperature (median value of the denaturation curve).

Table 2.
Example of a COMBO-FISH probe set for AMACR and some physical values considered in the selection of oligonucleotide stretches.

opening when probe and target are binding. TINA probes are oligonucleotides with additional anchoring molecules incorporated. Custom made oligonucleotide probes usually carry one dye molecule at one end or both ends each.

Depending on the base composition of the oligonucleotide probes, they can be designed in their 3′–5′ direction either for Watson–Crick binding (duplex forming probes result in complimentary probe-target double strands) or for Hoogsteen binding (triplex forming probes result in triple strands to homo-purine or homo-pyrimidine sequences as targets of the intact double strand) (**Figure 1**). COMBO-FISH probes targeting in Watson–Crick configuration are more flexible since they can be designed in a mixture of purine and pyrimidine bases. Hoogsteen binding probes use solely either purines or pyrimidines. It should mentioned that also exceptional (non-homo) Hoogsteen triples exist which can be incorporated into the probe design.

Due to the optical diffraction of a microscope lens, the point image of a fluorescence dye molecule spreads to an image of typically about 250 nm using a high numerical aperture lens. So the fluorescence of a probe combination within a target size less than typically about 250 kb merges into a homogeneous COMBO-FISH "spot". Typical examples are shown in **Figure 2**.

Detailed protocols for COMBO-FISH labeling of blood cells, fibroblasts, tumor culture cells, or tissue cells are described elsewhere [27, 29]. These protocols can be applied for duplex or triplex forming probe sets. COMBO-FISH for labeling of specific gene targets in cell nuclei has been described for several applications as for instance: The gene of the receptor tyrosine kinase 2 (HER2/NEU) [28, 34] (**Figure 2A** and **B**), the gene of the growth factor receptor-bound protein 7 (GRB7) [34], the breakpoint cluster region (BCR) on chromosome 22 [30], the ABL proto-oncogene 1 (ABL) on chromosome 9 [19, 30, 31], and T-box 1(TBX1) [33] (**Figure 2C** and **D**), the promotor region of the FMR1 gene [36] (**Figure 2E**) and the Alpha-Methylacyl-CoA Racemase coding gene (AMACR) on chromosome 5 [32] (**Table 2**; **Figure 2F**). Using the probe set for the ABL gene region and Spatially Modulated Illumination Microscopy [37], significant volume changes of the labeled regions were observed in cell nuclei of CML patients before and after medical treatment [35]. Beyond gene target labeling by probe sets of several

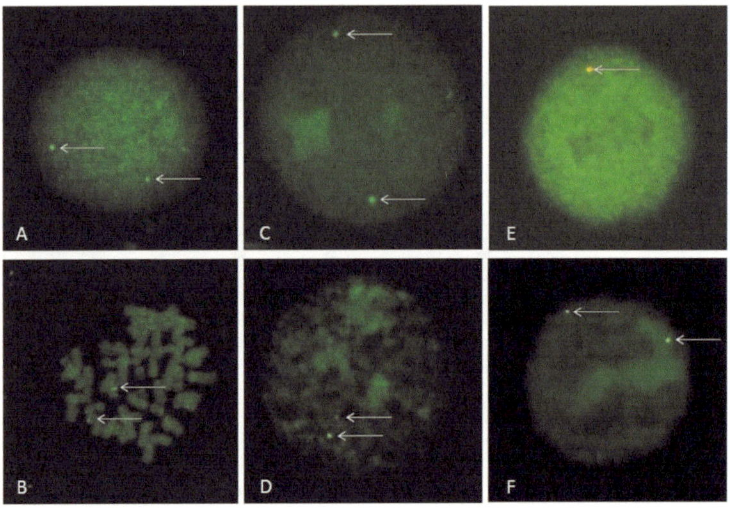

Figure 2.
Example fluorescence microscopy images of COMBO-FISH labeling (arrows) of gene targets: (A) HER2/NEU gene labeling in a cell nucleus and (B) on metaphase (combination of 18 oligonucleotide probes); (C) TBX1 gene labeling in a cell nucleus and (D) in an early stage of mitosis (combination of 15 oligonucleotide probes); (E) FMR1 promotor region labeling on chromosome X of a male cell nucleus (combination of 20 oligonucleotide probes); AMACR gene labeling in a cell nucleus (combination of 29 oligonucleotide probes; see ***Table*** *2). Note: With the exception of the nucleus in (E), no counterstain was applied.*

different probe-sequences co-localizing at a given target only, also unique probes were found that were specifically labeling either interspersed genome regions by one copy each or centromeres by multi-copies (see chapter 4). Such an 18mer oligonucleotide PNA probe repetitively binding on centromere 9 was micro-injected into lymphocyte cell nuclei under in vivo conditions. After further incubation of the labeled cells, the sample was fixed and subjected to microscopy. The results indicated that the probe material was binding to the target region in the nuclei before fixation [33].

3. COMBO-FISH probe sets for genes and breakpoint regions in oncology

Cancer cells are mutations of former "normal" cells. One reason for cancer cell malfunctions are over-expressions of genes, which are mainly caused by two reasons, either one gene is over-expressed or one gene is amplified and additionally to the original gene the copies also express. The latter frequently occurring in solid tumors leads to measureable copy number increases which can be used as diagnostic parameter in tumor biology and medicine. In contrast to solid tumors, blood cell tumors show structural aberration-like translocations in the early stages which can then be followed by numerical aberrations of larger chromosome parts or even whole chromosomes. Translocation chromosomes are resulting by fusion of two parts of different chromosomes that were broken very exactly at breakpoints within a certain breakpoint region; for example, for CML (chronic myeloid leukemia) a famous hallmark is the Philadelphia chromosome with the translocation ABL-BCR t(9,22)(q34,q11), in which a fusion of a part of the abl-region on chromosome 9 with part of the bcr-region on chromosome 22 takes place (for review [38]). Since the breaks occur very exactly at certain breakpoints the fusion region can be transcribed into a functioning protein that does normally not exist in a cell and that is involved in CML-induction.

Although appropriate target sites for homo-purine or homo-pyrimidine probes only make about a few percent of the genome, some prominent tumor genes and breakpoint regions can be specifically labeled by *uniquely co-localizing* sets of COMBO-FISH probes. Others can only be labeled by a set overlapping on neighboring regions. Probe sets for Her2/neu, abl, and bcr have been published elsewhere [29–31, 34]. In the following we will show further examples.

It has been observed that in various types of cancer such as breast, ovarian, and squamous cell cancer an amplification of 20q13 occurs. When analyzing such cancers it has been found that often the region which encodes ZNF217 is amplified and an increased expression of the specific region of ZNF217 has been observed. In some cases also neighboring gene encoding sequences are also amplified. It has to be mentioned that the detection of the copy number of ZNF217 can be done by standard FISH, but the shortest available sequence to detect ZNF217 has a length of about 245 kb [39], which means—compared to the length of ZNF217 of about 16 kb—that further amplifications within the probe-binding sequence might not have been visualized using this method. To further reduce the length of the detected target, a COMBO-FISH probe set was designed (**Table 3**). As a result, we obtained 25 oligonucleotide probes within a range of 133 kb. When reducing the number of sequences to 21 by removing the first and the last three probes the length of the considered DNA region can be downscaled to 91 kb.

The gene TP53 (sometimes called p53) encodes the "tumor protein 53" (P53). Its purpose is to maintain genomic stability and to control cell growth. Moreover, it is important for the induction of apoptosis and the coordination of repair processes. Labeling of this gene can be obtained by five COMBO-FISH probes only (**Table 4**).

Probe number	Beginning nucleotide number	
19,588	22,316,443	agggaggaaggagggaggaaggaagga
19,595	22,329,806	agagaaaagagagaaaa
19,600	22,332,226	agggaagaggaagagg
19,601	22,333,382	cctctctcttccctctccttcccctct
19,606	22,338,710	ttccttctttccttccttttctt
19,607	22,338,734	cttccttttctcccc
19,609	22,340,472	gagggaggagggagggaaaa
19,616	22,347,605	ggggaaagaaagaaa
19,623	22,352,916	tcttctcttttctttccttttcct
19,628	22,357,318	ctctttccccttctt
19,641	22,373,058	ggggagagaagaagg
19,643	22,373,175	ctttctcccttttccctcc
*19650	22,376,231	ccttttctcccctcccctcccctcccct
+19,659	22,389,995	cttctttcctcctttt
19,662	22,396,940	ctttcctccctctctct
19,665	22,403,663	ctcctccttcctcccct
19,671	22,407,703	ccctttcccctcctccct
19,674	22,410,694	ggaggggaagaagaggg
19,675	22,411,085	aaggagaagagaaagagag
19,676	22,411,601	gggagggggaggagggggggagg
19,677	22,412,039	aggagaggggaaaag
19,685	22,421,078	aggaggaaagagaggg
19,710	22,436,400	ggggaggggggaaaag
19,724	22,445,917	gagagagagagagagagagaagaaa
19,729	22,449,049	agaaagaaaagagaaagaagagaagag

*+, probe completely on ZNF217; *, probe partly on ZNF217.*

Table 3.
List of COMBO-FISH probe targets for ZNF217 and its surroundings (target sequences are written from left to right in the 5′-XXXX-3′ direction).

Probe number	Beginning nucleotide number	
7042	7,177,418	agaggaggggggagaag
7046	7,181,933	aggaagaggaaggaga
7067	7,193,067	cttctttecctccct
7068	7,193,145	aaagaaggggaggga
7069	7,193,288	ttttctctctetctcctcccctctc

Table 4.
List of COMBO-FISH probe targets for TP53 (target sequences are written from left to right in the 5′-XXXX-3′ direction).

The detection of 10 fluorochromes (dye molecules at both ends of each oligonucleotide probe) would require not only a sensitive microscope but also a background free preparation. Since in tumors P53 is inactivated (sometimes associated by a copy number loss of the gene, see, e.g., [40]), the protein MDM2 which can inactivate P53 when overexpressed can be investigated. In cells with an overexpression of MDM2 an extreme inactivation of the tumor suppressor protein can occur via binding of MDM2 to the transactivation domain of TP53. However, the treated gene, MDM2, does not contain sufficient homo-purine/homo-pyrimidine sequences so that a probe set has to be designed with an overlap on neighboring regions (**Table 5**).

Probe number	Beginning nucleotide number	
24,602	31,285,270	gaagagaagaaaggaga
24,603	31,287,071	aagagggaaggaaggg
24,605	31,288,864	cttttctcctccttct
24,608	31,292,189	aaggaagaggagaag
24,609	31,292,783	aagagagagaggggaggaaa
24,618	31,301,112	ctccctctcccccctccctcttttccctcctt
24,626	31,312,583	tctctcttcctcttctt
24,648	31,336,603	aaggaggaaggagaggaaaa
24,651	31,339,431	aagagaagggaggggaa
24,656	31,341,897	gggaaggaggagaaggggggagg
24,657	31,342,918	cttctctctctcccccc
24,659	31,344,079	gggagaagggaagga
+24,663	31,349,552	aaaaggaagggagaaag
+24,682	31,375,469	gggaaaaggaagaag
24,690	31,388,934	ttttctccccccttcccccttct
24,692	31,390,072	aagagggaggggaaaag
24,694	31,390,823	gggaaggggagggaaggggaggggag
*24695	31,390,850	ggaggaaagaagaaaaggaagggaaggggaggg
24,696	31,390,925	aggaagaggagaaggaaggaagaaaggaaagaaa
24,699	31,392,284	aaggaggaagagaaag
24,700	31,392,733	tttctcccttcttct
24,704	31,397,317	tttccttctccctttctct
24,706	31,398,270	ctttctttcctttcctctt
24,710	31,407,205	aagaggggaagggagag
24,724	31,422,982	aggaaaagaagaaaaga
24,726	31,425,374	aaagaaggagggaaa

*+, probe completely on MDM2; *, probe partly on MDM2.*

Table 5.
List of COMBO-FISH probe targets for MDM2 and its surroundings (target sequences are written from left to right in the 5′-XXXX-3′ direction).

CD44 is a receptor for hyaluronic acid, which plays an important role in cell migration, tumor growth and progression. Accumulating evidences have shown that the CD44 gene is abundantly expressed in cancer-initiating cells (CICs), and has thus been implicated as a CIC marker [41, 42] in several malignancies of hematopoietic and epithelial origin, including gastric cancer. Moreover, CD44 gene amplification was also found in gastric cancer. **Table 6** shows the targets for an appropriate CD44 gene probe set.

Fusion proteins originate from reciprocal translocations. Sets of oligonucleotides were designed in such a way that translocations get cognizable. There are two breakpoint regions—one on every chromosome. Therefore, four sets of oligonucleotides are needed: One before and after the breakpoint on the two chromosomes. For microscopy labeling with different colors is necessary; the sets of the first chromosome need to be labeled for instance with a red dye and the ones on the second chromosome, for instance, with a green dye. After hybridizing there are the following possible results: (a) Two red spots and two green spots are close together for each color, but the red ones are clearly separated from the green ones. This is the normal case without translocation. (b) There are two parts where one red and one green spot are next to each other. In this case the translocation has occurred: Both chromosomes broke at the major breakpoint and the wrong ends were joined. With four colors more details are visible. For example, when one color is visible on two locations, another breakpoint has been observed.

The minimum requirement for detecting clusters of homo-purine/homo-pyrimidine sequences on DNA is 6 oligonucleotides within a range of 250 kb. It is not necessary that the oligonucleotides are all located on the breakpoint regions itself. To get bright and emphasized signals, sets with 30 oligonucleotids each were designed for the following examples: ABL - BCR t(9,22)(q34,q11); AML1 - ETO t(8;21)(q22;q22); MYC - IGH t(8,14)(q24,q32); PML - RARA t(15,17)(q22,q21);PLZF - RARA t(11,17)(q23,q21). Since these lists would extend the article to an inacceptable size, the lists will be available from the authors on request.

4. COMBO-FISH with repetitively binding, unique single probes, and applications of super-resolution localization microscopy

The following chapter will focus on further novel developments of COMBO-FISH using probe sets of only one uniquely binding oligonucleotide [29] that binds repetitively to a given target like a centromere so that the merging fluorescence leads to a microscopic signal. In **Figure 3**, examples for centromere 9 [33] and 17 [34] are shown.

COMBO-FISH probes carrying one fluorochrome molecule at one end of each oligonucleotide are ideal nano-probes for Single Molecule Localization Microscopy [23, 24, 43] (SMLM) in order to analyze chromatin structure and architecture on the nano-scale in subchromosomal regions of cell nuclei [32, 43–47].

As an example, multiple copies of a repetitive probe for a tri-nucleotide expansion region were hybridized and analyzed quantitatively in cells with Fragile-X syndrome (FXS) or Martin-Bell-Syndrome. FXS belongs to the group of the so-called "trinucleotide repeat expansion disorders" consisting of the expansion of a trinucleotide frequency ((CGG)n-expansion) in the 5′ untranslated region of the Fragile-X Mental Retardation 1 gene (FMR1) on the X-chromosome. The enlargement of the CGG triplet-repeat results in a deactivation of the FMR1 gene and mental retardation of the patient. Multiplets of 6 trinucleotide units ($(CGG)_6$ or $(CCG)_6$ probes) were synthesized showing high specificity to the (CGG)-repeat expansion of the FMR1 gene; thereby a minimum of accessory binding sites were found due to the 6-times

Probe number	Beginning nucleotide number	
24,971	35,103,408	gaaggggagaaggaggaaaggggaaggaaaggag
−24,972	35,108,828	gagggagggagagaaa
24,973	35,109,919	aagagggggaggggaa
24,975	35,112,662	agagagaggggagaggagagaaa
24,977	35,119,179	ctccctccttcctcctc
24,978	35,120,540	ttttcctccctctccc
24,980	35,121,359	ctccttctccctttt
−24,981	35,122,451	tctctctttctctttctctctctctc
24,982	35,123,378	gggggggaagaggag
24,984	35,126,758	agggagagaaagaaa
24,985	35,129,005	tccttttcccttcct
24,986	35,132,494	tttcttcccctctct
−24,987	35,135,378	cctctctcctttctte
−24,988	35,136,463	aggaaggagagaaagagag
24,991	35,139,280	gaaagggaaaaggaaag
−24,992	35,139,595	agagagagggagaaag
24,993	35,140,078	aaaaggggaggaaag
−24,994	35,141,641	tctctttccctctct
24,996	35,146,244	tcttcttttctcctttt
−24,998	35,147,116	tcttcctccctccctctctcc
24,999	35,147,168	tctccttcttcctcttt
25,004	35,151,365	ccttttctctctccc
25,013	35,169,216	aaaggggggaagaggg
25,014	35,173,890	tcttctctcctcccccc
25,019	35,181,667	ggggaaagagaagaa
−25,021	35,185,117	ccctctccctcctccc
25,022	35,185,516	aaggagaaagagaagg
25,026	35,192,486	agaaagaagaagaaaag
25,027	35,192,612	ccctctcccctccctctctccctcc
−25,028	35,192,661	cttcctttctcttct

−, probes are excluded since they form secondary clusters.

Table 6.
List of COMBO-FISH probe targets for the CD44 gene (target sequences are written from left to right in the 5′-XXXX-3′ direction).

repetition. Considering the probe length of six trinucleotide units together with one dye molecule at one end, the results of SMLM indicated small chromatin loops for the expansion region rearranging chromatin on the nanoscale so that a deactivation could be explained by geometric reasons in the genome architecture [36].

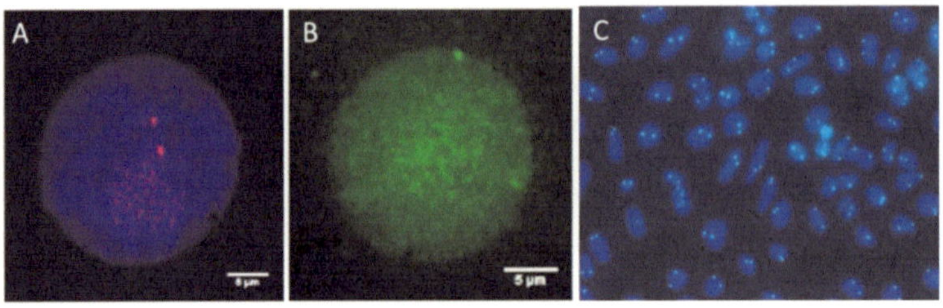

Figure 3.
Example fluorescence microscopy images of COMBO-FISH labeling of centromere targets: (A) centromere 17 labeling in a lymphocyte cell nucleus with the repetitively binding probe (Alexa647-5′-cttctgtcttctttttata-3′) and (B) with the repetitively binding probe (Alexa488-5′-tataaaaagaagacagaag-3′). In (C) an overview image of centromere 9 labeling in lymphocyte cell nuclei with the repetitively binding probe (Alexa546-5′-aatcaacccgagtgcaat-3′) is shown indicating a hybridization efficiency better than 90%.

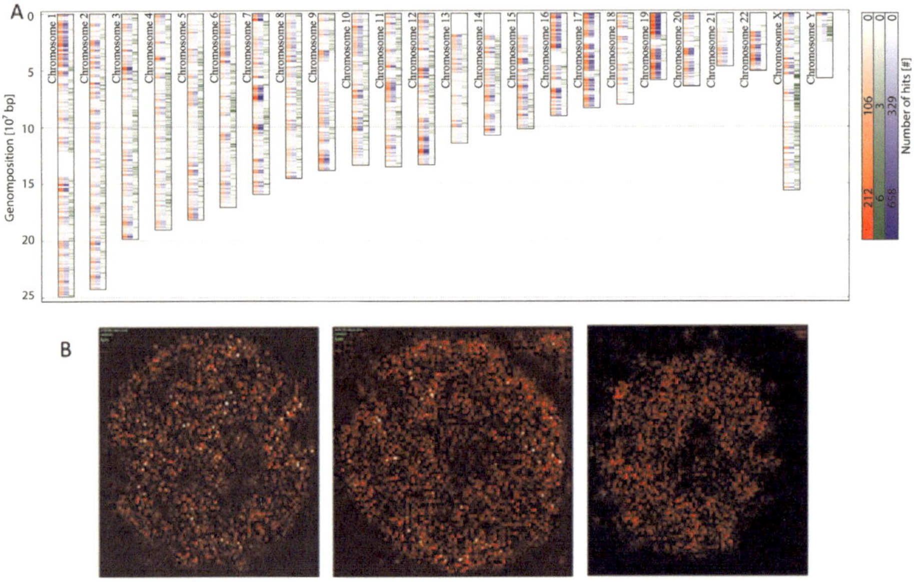

Figure 4.
(A) ALU-distribution along the genome: The intensity of the bars indicates the frequency within a 500 kb section of the given chromosome. Red: Position of the designed 17mer ALU probe. The sequence associated with the ALU probe appears in the entire genome at different frequency densities. Blue: Corresponding positions of the ALU consensus sequence. The number of emergence of the 17mer probe sequence was compared with the density of the ALU consensus sequence by using the program "Repeatmasker" [50]. Green: Distribution of a selected 17mer from the L1 element. Although this 17mer appears very often in the genome, the frequency density is significantly different from the selected ALU consensus 17mer. (B) Examples of SMLM images of cell nuclei after COMBO-FISH labeling with the 17mer ALU probe. Note: (A) was originally published under CC BY license in [48].

Although established programs for the design of COMBO-FISH probes and probe sets were available [20, 26], novel so-called alignment-free investigations of k-mers, their frequencies and their positioning along the nucleotide sequence of a chromosome [48, 49] have found oligonucleotide probes that uniquely bind in a given repetition rate to chromatin sequences repetitively occurring as interspersed motives [29]. New generations of specific COMBO-FISH probes were elucidated against SINEs (Short Interspersed Nuclear Elements, e.g., ALU elements [32, 48, 50], **Figure 4**), LINEs (Long Interspersed Nuclear Elements, e.g., L1 [32]), or centromeres [44]. With

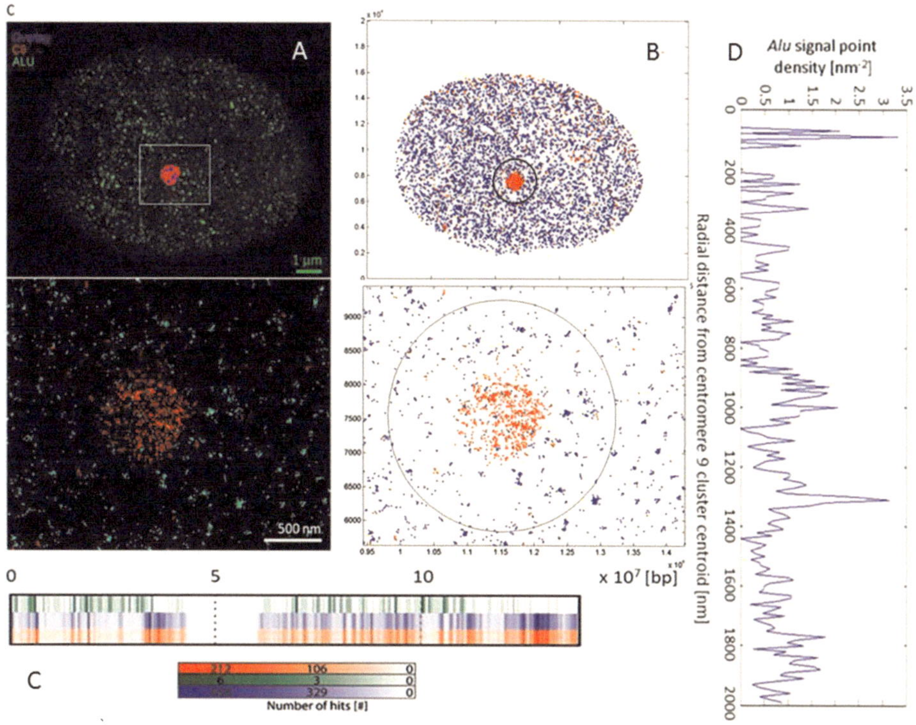

Figure 5.
(A) SMLM overlay image of Alu densities (green), a centromere 9 points cluster (red), and overlaying regions (blue). Note: Only one image plane (no projection) is shown, where one centromere 9 is located. A magnified point coordinate representation of the white box is shown below. (B)–(D) Estimates of chromosome 9 architecture by its centromere and genomic Alu. (B) Plot of the raw point matrix obtained from SMLM data of (A). A circular approximation of a chromosome 9 territory (black circle) modeled from the theoretical distribution of Alu elements (blue dots) around the chromosome 9 centromere (red dots). Lower image: Magnification of the region of interest in the upper image. (C) Idiogram of chromosome 9 showing the positional distribution of Alu probe binding sites (red), Alu consensus sequences (blue), and binding sites of a probe against genomic L1 elements (green). (D) The radial distribution of Alu signal points around a centromere 9 cluster centroid averaged over 38 centromere 9 clusters. Note: These figures were originally published under CC BY license in [32].

these probes, first evaluations of the spatial organization of chromosome 9 were calculated (**Figure 5**) [32].

Using quantitative SMLM, the in such a way designed ALU COMBO-FISH probe has also been successfully applied in extending the standard methods of biological dosimetry, which aims at reconstructing or estimating from chromosome aberrations the dose from former radiation exposure [48, 50]. In addition, a novel improved preparation protocol circumvents any heat treatment for target denaturation so that mixed purine–pyrimidine probes can be used, that usually undergo Watson–Crick double-strand pairing (**Figure 1**). This so-called low-temperature protocol is the prerequisite to combine oligonucleotide-based COMBO-FISH and immunofluorescence staining by means of specific antibodies [29, 48].

5. Conclusion

COMBO-FISH offers a highly variable toolbox of labeling combinations and strategies for chromatin architecture and bio-medical research. Here we have introduced three strategies: (a) Design of a COMBO-FISH probe set which consists of several oligonucleotide probes that *specifically co-localize* at a given genome target as for instance, a tumor-relevant gene that could be involved in gene copy number changes or tumor-inducing translocations. (b) Design of a COMBO-FISH probe set which consists of one oligonucleotide probe which *in many copies specifically co-localize* at a given genome target as for instance a centromere. (c) Design of a COMBO-FISH probe set which consists of one oligonucleotide probe that *uniquely occurs* at several given repetitively occurring genome targets only as for instance SINEs or LINEs. The efficiency of the probe set can be further enhanced by incorporating structural [51–53] and dynamical parameters determined by molecular dynamics simulations (e.g., AMBER [54–56], GROMOS [57, 58], CHARMM [59, 60]) into the probe design, which we currently investigate.

In combination with super-resolution localization microscopy and novel tools of data evaluation and interpretation by geometric and topological algorithms [61–64] COMBO-FISH probes offer new perspectives in understanding the reaction of chromatin as a system as a whole during gene expression, proliferation, or stress response [47].

Acknowledgements

The authors thank former and present team members, Wilhelm von Rosenberg, Laura Doll, Jens Rösler, Stefan Stein, Michael Stuhlmüller, Jin-Ho Lee, Florence Laure Djikimi Tchetgna, Matthias Krufczik, Aaron Sievers, and Jutta Schwarz-Finsterle at the Kirchhoff-Institute of Physics, Heidelberg University for images taken from their theses and publications.

Conflict of interest

The authors declare no conflict of interest.

Author details

Michael Hausmann* and Eberhard Schmitt
Kirchhoff-Institute for Physics, Heidelberg University, Heidelberg, Germany

*Address all correspondence to: hausmann@kip.uni-heidelberg.de

References

[1] Boveri T. Die Blastomerenkerne von Ascaris megalocephala und die Theorie der Chromosomenindividualität. Archiv für Experimentelle Zellforschung. 1909; **3**:181-268

[2] Rabl C. Über Zellteilung. Gegenbaurs Morphologisches Jahrbuch. 1885;**10**: 214-330

[3] Cremer T, Cremer C. Chromosome territories, nuclear architecture and gene regulation in mammalian cells. Nature Reviews. Genetics. 2001;**2**:292-301

[4] Ma T, Chen L, Shi M, Niu J, Zhang X, Yang X, et al. Developing novel methods to image and visualize 3D genomes. Cell Biology and Toxicology. 2018;**34**: 367-380

[5] Hausmann M, Lee J-H, Hildenbrand G. 3D DNA FISH for analyses of chromatin-nuclear architecture. In: Tollefsbol T, editor. Epigenetics Methods. Vol. 18. Amsterdam: Academic Press, Elsevier; 2020. pp. 399-418. DOI: doi.org/10.1016/B978-0-12-819414-0.00020-3

[6] Wolf D, Rauch J, Hausmann M, Cremer C. Comparison of the thermal denaturation behaviour of DNA-solutions and chromosome preparations in suspension. Biophysical Chemistry. 1999;**81**:207-221

[7] Rauch J, Wolf D, Hausmann M, Cremer C. The influence of formamide on thermal denaturation profiles of DNA and metaphase chromosomes in suspensions. Zeitschrift für Naturforschung. Section C. 2000;**55**: 737-746

[8] Bridger JM, Volpi EV, editors. Fluorescence In Situ Hybridization (FISH) – Protocols and Applications. Springer, New York, Dordrecht, Heidelberg, London: Humana Press; 2010

[9] Egholm M, Buchardt O, Christensen L, Behrens C, Freier SM, Driver DA, et al. PNA hybridizes to complementary oligonucleotides obeying the Watson-Crick hydrogen-bonding rules. Nature. 1993;**365**:566-568

[10] Matera AG, Ward DC. Oligonucleotide probes for the analysis of specific repetitive DNA sequences by fluorescence in situ hybridization. Human Molecular Genetics. 1992;**1**: 535-539

[11] Beliveau BJ, Boettiger AN, Avendano MS, Jungmann R, McCole RB, Joyce EF, et al. Single-molecule super-resolution imaging of chromosomes and in situ haplotype visualization using Oligopaint FISH probes. Nature Communications. 2015;**6**:7147

[12] Beliveau BJ, Joyce EF, Apostolopoulos N, Yilmaz F, Fonseka CY, McCole RB, et al. Versatile design and synthesis platform for visualizing genomes with Oligopaint FISH probes. Proceedings of the National Academy of Sciences of the United States of America. 2012;**109**:21301-21306

[13] Boyle S, Rodesch MJ, Halvensleben HA, Jeddeloh JA, Bickmore WA. Fluorescence in situ hybridization with high-complexity repeat-free oligonucleotide probes generated by massively parallel synthesis. Chromosome Research. 2011; **19**:901-909

[14] Yamada NA, Rector LS, Tsang P, Carr E, Scheffer A, Sederberg MC, et al. Visualization of fine-scale genomic structure by oligonucleotide-based

high-resolution FISH. Cytogenetic and Genome Research. 2010;**132**:248-254

[15] Winkler R, Perner B, Rapp A, Durm M, Cremer C, Greulich KO, et al. Labelling quality and chromosome morphology after low temperature FISH analysed by scanning far-field and scanning near-field optical microscopy. Journal of Microscopy. 2003;**209**:23-33

[16] Dobruck J, Darzynkiewicz Z. Chromatin condensation and sensitivity of DNA in situ to denaturation during cell cycle and apoptosis – a confocal microscopy study. Micron. 2001;**32**: 645-652

[17] Genet MD, Cartwright IM, Kato TA. Direct DNA and PNA probe binding to telomeric regions without classical in situ hybridization. Molecular Cytogenetics. 2013;**6**:42

[18] Cremer C, Hausmann M, Cremer T (1998) Markierung von Nukleinsäuren mit speziellen Probengemischen. German Patent DE 198 06 962 A1.

[19] Hausmann M, Winkler R, Hildenbrand G, Finsterle J, Weisel A, Rapp A, et al. COMBO-FISH: Specific labelling of nondenatured chromatin targets by computer-selected DNA oligonucleotide probe combinations. BioTechniques. 2003;**35**: 564-577

[20] Schmitt E, Wagner J, Hausmann M. Combinatorial selection of short triplex forming oligonucleotides for fluorescence in situ hybridisation COMBO-FISH. Journal of Computer Science. 2012;**3**:328-334

[21] Felsenfeld G, Davies DR, Rich A. Formation of a three-stranded polynucleotide molecule. Journal of the American Chemical Society. 1957;**79**: 2023-2024

[22] Felsenfeld G, Rich A. Studies on the formation of two and three stranded polynucleotides. Biochimica et Biophysica Acta. 1957;**26**:457-468

[23] Lemmer P, Gunkel M, Baddeley D, Kaufmann R, Urich A, Weiland Y, et al. SPDM – light microscopy with single molecule resolution at the nanoscale. Applied Physics B: Lasers and Optics. 2008;**93**:1-12

[24] Cremer C, Kaufmann R, Gunkel M, Pres S, Weiland Y, Müller P, et al. Super-resolution imaging of biological nanostructures by Spectral Precision Distance Microscopy (SPDM). Reviews in Biotechnology. 2011;**6**: 1037-1051

[25] Eberle JP, Rapp A, Krufczik M, Eryilmaz M, Gunkel M, Erfle H, et al. Super-resolution microscopy techniques and their potential for applications in radiation biophysics. In: Erfle H, editor. Super-resolution Microscopy – Methods and Protocols, Methods in Molecular Biology. Vol. 1663. Totowa, New Jersey: Springer; 2017. pp. 1-13

[26] Kepper N, Schmitt E, Lesnussa M, Weiland Y, Eussen HB, Grosveld F, et al. Visualization, analysis, and design of COMBO-FISH probes in the Grid-based GLOBE 3D genome platform. In: Solomonides T, Blanquer I, Breton V, Glatard T, Legré Y, editors. Healthgrid Applications and Core Technologies: Proceedings of HealthGrid, Studies in Health Technology and Informatics. Vol. 159. Amsterdam: IOS Press; 2010. pp. 171-180

[27] Schmitt E, Schwarz-Finsterle J, Stein S, Boxler C, Müller P, Mokhir A, et al. Combinatorial oligo FISH: Directed labelling of specific genome domains in differentially fixed cell material and live cells. In: Bidger JM, Volpi EV, editors. Fluorescence In Situ Hybrdization,

Methods in Molecular Biology. Vol. 659. Totowa, New Jersey: Springer; 2010. pp. 185-202

[28] Zeller D, Kepper N, Hausmann M, Schmitt E. Sequential and structural biophysical aspects of combinatorial oligo-FISH in Her2/Neu breast cancer diagnostics. IFMBE Proceedings. 2013; **38**:82-85

[29] Hausmann M, Lee J-H, Sievers A, Krufczik M, Hildenbrand G. COMBinatorial Oligonucleotide FISH (COMBO-FISH) with uniquely binding repetitive DNA probes. In: Hancock R, editor. The Nucleus, Methods in Molecular Biology. Vol. 2175. Totowa, New Jersey: Springer; 2020. pp. 65-77

[30] Schwarz-Finsterle J, Stein S, Großmann C, Schmitt E, Schneider H, Trakhtenbrot L, et al. COMBO-FISH for focussed fluorescence labelling of gene domains: 3D-analysis of the genome architecture of abl and bcr in human blood cells. Cell Biology International. 2005;**29**:1038-1046

[31] Schwarz-Finsterle J, Stein S, Großmann C, Schmitt E, Trakhtenbrot L, Rechavi G, et al. Comparison of triplehelical COMBO-FISH and standard FISH by means of quantitative microscopic image analysis of abl/bcr genome organisation. Journal of Biochemical and Biophysical Methods. 2007;**70**:397-406

[32] Lee J-H, Laure Djikimi Tchetgna F, Krufczik M, Schmitt E, Cremer C, Bestvater F, et al. COMBO-FISH: A versatile tool beyond standard FISH to study chromatin organization by fluorescence light microscopy. OBM Genetics. 2019;**3**(1):064; pp. 28. DOI: 10.21926/obm.genet.1901064

[33] Nolte O, Müller M, Häfner B, Knemeyer J-P, Stöhr K, Wolfrum J, et al. Novel singly labelled probes for identification of microorganisms, detection of antibiotic resistance genes and mutations, and tumor diagnosis (SMART PROBES). In: Popp J, Strehle M, editors. Biophotonics. Weinheim: Wiley-VCH; 2006. pp. 167-230

[34] Müller P, Rößler J, Schwarz-Finsterle J, Pedersen EB, Géci I, Schmitt E, et al. PNA-COMBO-FISH: From combinatorial probe design in silico to vitality compatible, specific labelling of gene targets in cell nuclei. Experimental Cell Research. 2016; **345**:51-59

[35] Grossmann C, Schwarz-Finsterle J, Schmitt E, Birk U, Hildenbrand G, Cremer C, et al. Variations of the spatial fluorescence distribution in ABL gene chromatin domains measured in blood cell nuclei by SMI microscopy after COMBO-FISH labelling. In: Méndez-Vilas A, Díaz Álvarez J, editors. Microscopy: Science, Technology, Applications and Education. Vol. 1. Badajoz, España: Formatex Research Center; 2010. pp. 688-695

[36] Stuhlmüller M, Schwarz-Finsterle J, Fey E, Lux J, Bach M, Cremer C, et al. In situ optical sequencing and nano-structure analysis of a trinucleotide expansion region by localization microscopy after specific COMBO-FISH labelling. Nanoscale. 2015;**7**:17938-17946

[37] Hausmann M, Hildenbrand G, Schwarz-Finsterle J, Birk U, Schneider H, Cremer C, et al. New technologies measure genome domains – high resolution microscopy and novel labeling procedures enable 3-D studies of the functional architecture of gene domains in cell nuclei. Biophotonics International. 2005;**12**(10):34-37

[38] Senapati J, Sasaki K. Chromosomal instability in chronic myeloid leukemia: Mechanistic insights and effects.

Cancers. 2022;**14**(10):2533. DOI: 10.3390/cancers 14102533

[39] Cytocell Ltd ZNF217 Amplification LPS 005, Available from: http://www.cytocell.co.uk/products/aquarius/pathology/ZNF217-probe. 2012

[40] Albrecht B, Hausmann M, Zitzelsberger H, Stein H, Siewert JR, Hopt U, et al. Array-based comparative genomic hybridization for the detection of DNA sequence copy number changes in Barrett's adenocarcinoma. The Journal of Pathology. 2004;**203**:780-788

[41] Chen C, Zhao S, Karnad A, Freeman JW. The biology and role of CD44 in cancer progression: Therapeutic implications. Journal of Hematology & Oncology. 2018;**11**:64. DOI: 10.1186/s13045-018-0605-5

[42] Xu H, Niu M, Yuan X, Wu K, Liu A. CD44 as a tumor biomarker and therapeutic target. Experimental Hematology & Oncology. 2020;**9**:36. DOI: doi.org/10.1186/s40164-020-00192-0

[43] Müller P, Weiland Y, Kaufmann R, Gunkel M, Hillebrandt S, Cremer C, Hausmann M. Analysis of fluorescent nanostructures in biological systems by means of Spectral Position Determination Microscopy (SPDM). In: Méndez-Vilas A, editor. Current Microscopy Contributions to Advances in Science and Technology. Badajoz, España: Formatex Research Center; 2021;**1**:3-12

[44] Müller P, Schmitt E, Jacob A, Hoheisel J, Kaufmann R, Cremer C, et al. COMBO-FISH enables high precision localization microscopy as a prerequisite for nanostructure analysis of genome loci. International Journal of Molecular Sciences. 2010;**11**:4094-4105

[45] Krigerts J, Salmina K, Freivalds T, Zayakin P, Rumnieks F, Inashkina I, et al. Differentiating breast cancer cells reveal early large-scale genome regulation by pericentric domains. Biophysical Journal. 2021;**120**:711-724. https://doi.org/10.1016/j.bpj.2021.01.002

[46] Erenpreisa J, Krigerts J, Salmina K, Gerashchenko BI, Freivalds T, Kurg R, et al. Heterochromatin networks: topology, dynamics, and function (a working hypothesis). Cell. 2021;**10**:1582. https://doi.org/10.3390/cells10071582

[47] Hausmann M, Hildenbrand G, Pilarczyk G. Networks and islands of genome nano-architecture and their potential relevance for radiation biology (A hypothesis and experimental verification hints). In: Kloc M, Kubiak JZ, editors. Nuclear, Chromosomal, and Genomic Architecture in Biology and Medicine. In press. Berlin, Heidelberg: Springer; 2022

[48] Krufczik M, Sievers A, Hausmann A, Lee J-H, Hildenbrand G, Schaufler W, et al. Combining low temperature fluorescence DNA-hybridization, immunostaining, and super-resolution localization microscopy for nano-structure analysis of ALU elements and their influence on chromatin structure. International Journal of Molecular Sciences. 2017;**18**:1005. DOI: 10.3390/ijms18051005

[49] Sievers A, Bosiek K, Bisch M, Dreessen C, Riedel J, Froß P, et al. Kmer content, correlation and position analysis of genome DNA sequences for identification of function and evolutionary features. Genes. 2017;**8**:122. DOI: 10.3390/genes8040122

[50] Hausmann M, Ilić N, Pilarczyk G, Lee J-H, Logeswaran A, Borroni AP, et al. Challenges for super-resolution localization microscopy and biomolecular fluorescent nano-probing

in cancer research. International Journal of Molecular Sciences. 2017;**18**:2066. DOI: 10.3390/ijms18102066

[51] Markham NR, Zuker M. DINAMelt web server for nucleic acid melting prediction. Nucleic Acids Research. 2005; **33**:W577-W581. DOI: 10.1093/nar/gki591

[52] Zuker M. Mfold web server for nucleic acid folding and hybridization prediction. Nucleic Acids Research. 2003;**31**: 3406-3415. DOI: 10.1093/nar/gkg595

[53] Mathews DH, Turner DH. Prediction of RNA secondary structure by free energy minimization. Current Opinion in Structural Biology. 2006;**16**:270-278. DOI: doi.org/10.1016/j.sbi.2006.05.010

[54] General information on: https://ambermd.org/

[55] Case DA, Cheatham TE, Darden T, Gohlke H, Luo R, Merz KM Jr, et al. The AMBER biomolecular simulation programs. Journal of Computational Chemistry. 2005;**26**(16):1668-1688. DOI: 10.1002/jcc.20290

[56] Salomon-Ferrer R, Case DA, Walker RC. An overview of the Amber biomolecular simulation package. WIREs Computational Molecular Science. 2013;**3**:198-210. DOI: 10.1002/wcms.112

[57] General information on: http://www.gromos.net/

[58] Schmid N, Christ CD, Christen M, Eichenberger AP, van Gunsteren WF. Architecture, implementation and parallelisation of the GROMOS Software for biomolecular simulation. Computer Physics Communications. 2012;**183**: 890-903

[59] General information on: https://www.charmm.org/, https://academiccharmm.org/

[60] Hynninen A, Crowley MF. New faster CHARMM molecular dynamics engine. Journal of Computational Chemistry. 2014;**35**:406-413. DOI: 10.1002/jcc.23501

[61] Hofmann A, Krufczik M, Heermann DW, Hausmann M. Using persistent homology as a new approach for super-resolution localization microscopy data analysis and classification of γH2AX foci/clusters. International Journal of Molecular Sciences. 2018;**19**:2263. DOI: 10.3390/ijms19082263

[62] Hausmann M, Neitzel C, Bobkova E, Nagel D, Hofmann A, Chramko T, et al. Single molecule localization microscopy analyses of DNA-repair foci and clusters detected along particle damage tracks. Frontiers of Physics. 2020;**8**:578662. DOI: 10.3389/fphy.2020.578662

[63] Hausmann M, Falk M, Neitzel C, Hofmann A, Biswas A, Gier T, et al. Elucidation of the clustered nano-architecture of radiation-induced DNA damage sites and surrounding chromatin in cancer cells: A single molecule localization microscopy approach. International Journal of Molecular Sciences. 2021;**22**:3636. DOI: doi.org/10.3390/ijms22073636

[64] Hahn H, Neitzel C, Kopečná O, Heermann DW, Falk M, Hausmann M. Topological analysis of γH2AX and MRE11 clusters detected by localization microscopy during X-ray-induced DNA double-strand break repair. Cancers. 2021;**13**:5561. https://doi.org/10.3390/cancers13215561

Chapter 5

The Natural Antisense Transcript-Targeted Regulation Technology Using Sense Oligonucleotides and Its Application

Mikio Nishizawa, Tetsuya Okuyama and Richi Nakatake

Abstract

Natural antisense transcripts (NATs or AS transcripts) are frequently transcribed from many eukaryotic genes and post-transcriptionally regulate gene expression. The AS transcript is classified as noncoding RNA and acts as a regulatory RNA in concert with RNA-binding proteins that bind to cis-controlling elements on the mRNA, microRNAs, and drugs. The AS transcript that overlaps with mRNA regulates mRNA stability by interacting with mRNA, and the network of mRNAs, AS transcripts, microRNAs, and RNA-binding proteins finely tunes the output of gene regulation, i.e., mRNA levels. We found that single-stranded 'sense' oligonucleotides corresponding to an mRNA sequence decreased the mRNA levels by interfering with the mRNA-AS transcript interactions of several genes, such as inducible nitric oxide synthase (*iNOS*) and interferon-alpha1 (*IFN-A1*) genes. In contrast, AntagoNAT oligonucleotides, which are complementary to AS transcripts, are sense oligonucleotides when they overlap with mRNA, but they increase the levels of specific mRNAs. Collectively, the sense oligonucleotide is a powerful tool for decreasing or increasing mRNA levels. The natural antisense transcript-targeted regulation (NATRE) technology using sense oligonucleotides is a method with a unique modality for modulating cytosolic mRNA levels and may be used to treat human diseases in which AS transcripts are involved.

Keywords: antisense transcript, noncoding RNA, microRNA, mRNA stability, sense oligonucleotide, locked nucleic acid

1. Introduction

The transcripts whose sequences are complementary to those of mRNA have been reported in many genes regardless of species, from bacteria to mammals. Because protein is encoded by mRNA, whose sequence is the same as the sense strand of a gene, i.e., double-stranded DNA, the transcript has been called a natural antisense transcript (NAT or AS transcript) [1, 2]. The AS transcripts do not code for proteins or only short peptides and are classified as one class of noncoding RNA (ncRNA). Accumulating genome-wide transcriptome analyses have demonstrated that natural antisense transcripts are transcribed from many eukaryotic genes [3]. HUGO proposed the nomenclature of human gene symbols for natural antisense transcripts *AS* (suffix) [4]. In this chapter, we use 'AS transcript' as a natural antisense transcript.

In contrast, classical types of ncRNA species, such as ribosomal RNA (rRNA), transfer RNA (tRNA), small nuclear RNA (snRNA), and small nucleolar RNA (snoRNA), are well known and have definite functions in gene expression. These classical ncRNAs do not overlap mRNAs. Among other ncRNA species, microRNA (miRNA or miR), which is 20–23 nucleotides (nt) in the length, was found in nematodes and mammals. This very short ncRNA species, which is complementary to the 3′-untranslated region (3′UTR) of several mRNAs, inhibits translation and induces mRNA degradation [5]. Therefore, microRNA hybridizes with mRNA to regulate its functions.

Furthermore, long ncRNAs (lncRNAs), which are more than 200 nt long [6], were found. At first, their functions were unclear, but it has gradually been revealed that these lncRNAs are involved in gene expression [7]. To date, huge number of lncRNA sequences have been reported by RNA-seq analysis and deposited in public databases, such as LNCipedia 5 (human lncRNA transcripts) [8]. Nowadays, ncRNA species, including miRNA, and lncRNAs, are known as *regulatory RNAs* [9].

Many studies have demonstrated that the AS transcript, one class of lncRNA, is involved in various steps during gene expression [7]. When focusing on the AS transcript that overlaps with an mRNA, this type of AS transcript interacts with mRNA and plays an important role in gene expression, especially at post-transcriptional levels [1, 2]. Interestingly, most AS transcripts are transcribed at low levels [1, 2]. The analyses and application of AS transcripts are summarized by the reviews, for example, see [1, 2, 10].

During our functional analyses of AS transcripts, we found the mRNA-AS transcript interactions that regulate mRNA stability (described later). Although conventional methods, i.e., antisense and short interference RNA (siRNA) technologies [11, 12] were available for the analyses of AS transcript functions [13], we first used synthetic sense oligonucleotides that are complementary to the AS transcript. We found that sense oligonucleotides resulted in decreases in cytoplasmic mRNA levels, which may be applied to 'knockdown of mRNA.'

Here, our method to regulate mRNA levels based on the mRNA-AS transcript interactions is described, and the application of this technology to treat disease is discussed.

2. Natural antisense transcripts that overlap with mRNAs

2.1 Structures of natural antisense transcripts

The AS transcript is frequently transcribed from inducible genes [14]. Our previous studies showed that an AS transcript harbors an overlapping sequence with 3′UTR of an mRNA [14]. Such a 3′UTR possesses a few AU-rich elements (AREs), which may be involved in mRNA stability because AREs may be the targets of miRNAs and RNA-binding proteins [15, 16]. Interestingly, the location of AREs in the 3′UTR of *iNOS* mRNA is conserved among species (rat, mouse, and human) [17, 18].

The sizes of AS transcripts are variable and show a smear pattern or discrete bands in Northern blot analysis. The former example is AS transcripts that are transcribed from rat inducible nitric oxide synthase (*iNOS*, *NOS2*) gene, and the size is ranging from 600 to 1000 nt (**Figure 1**) [19]. iNOS catalyzes the production of the inflammatory mediator nitric oxide (NO). iNOS is induced by various inflammatory stimuli; interleukin (IL)-1beta to hepatocytes and bacterial lipopolysaccharide (LPS) to macrophages [17, 18].

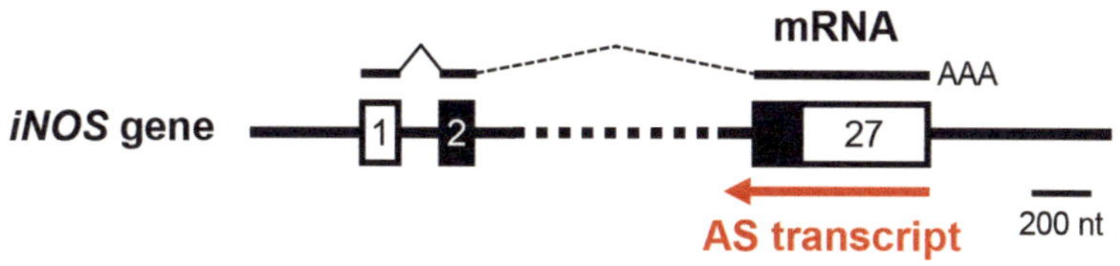

Figure 1.
mRNA and AS transcripts transcribed from the inducible nitric oxide synthase (iNOS) gene. The rat iNOS gene is schematically depicted. The iNOS gene consists of 27 exons, and the AS transcript overlaps with the exon 27, which includes the 3′UTR (white box) of the mRNA. The iNOS mRNA harbors AREs in its 3′UTR. The iNOS AS transcript starts at the end of exon 27 and stops at various sites, resulting in various sizes of the transcripts, which do not harbor a poly(A) tail. Figure reproduced with modification from [19] with permission.

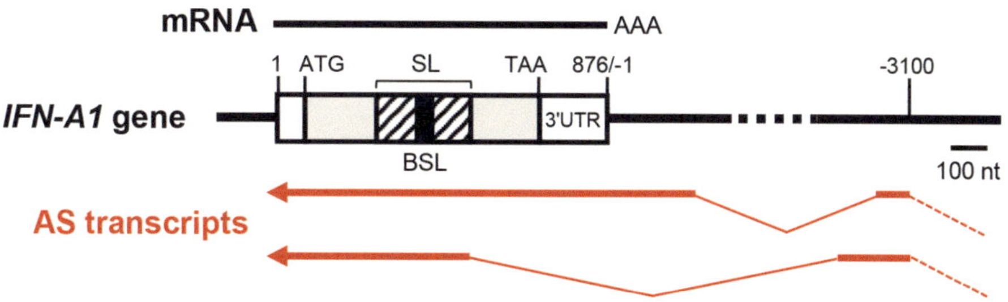

Figure 2.
mRNA and AS transcripts transcribed from interferon alpha1 (IFN-A1) gene. The human IFN-A1 gene consists of a single exon, which encodes IFN-alpha1 [20]. The coding sequence (from ATG to TAA) gives conserved stem-loop structures in the IFN-A1 mRNA, i.e., stem-loops (SL) and bulged-stem loop (BSL) [21]. These structures are responsible for chromosome region maintenance 1 (CRM1)-dependent nuclear export of IFN-A1 mRNA [21]. The IFN-A1 mRNA harbors AREs in its 3′UTR. Two AS transcripts are shown, both of which are spliced and harbor poly(A) tails. Nucleotides are numbered from the transcription initiation site. Figure reproduced with modification from [20] with permission.

The latter examples are about 4-kilobase (kb) AS transcript that is transcribed from the human interferon-alpha1 (*IFN-A1*) gene (**Figure 2**) [20]. *IFN-A1* gene encodes the cytokine IFN-alpha1 and is one subset of human *IFN-A* genes, which consist of 13 subsets [22]. Viral infection induces IFN-alpha1, a member of the type I interferon family, which is a main innate immunity response. AS transcripts are also transcribed from other subtypes of *IFN-A* genes [23].

Another example is the AS transcript from the rat tumor necrosis factor-alpha (*Tnf*) gene, which is about 2.5-kb long [24]. AS transcripts are transcribed from many genes that are involved in inflammation, such as mRNAs that encode alpha subunit (p19) of IL-23 (IL-23A), chemokine (C-C motif) ligand 2 (CCL2), chemokine (C-X_3-C) motif ligand 1 (CX3CL1), p65 and p50 subunits of nuclear factor kappaB (NF-kappaB) [14]. Additionally, AS transcript is transcribed from the human gene encoding ephrin type A receptor 2 (EPHA2), which is a receptor tyrosine kinase whose over-expression is observed in various cancers [25, 26].

2.2 mRNA-AS transcript interactions and mRNA stability

2.2.1 iNOS mRNA-AS transcript interaction

When the AS transcript overlaps with the relevant mRNA, the interaction between the AS transcript and mRNA is expected. Indeed, the AS transcript is transcribed from the rat *iNOS* gene and interacts with and stabilizes the *iNOS* mRNA [19].

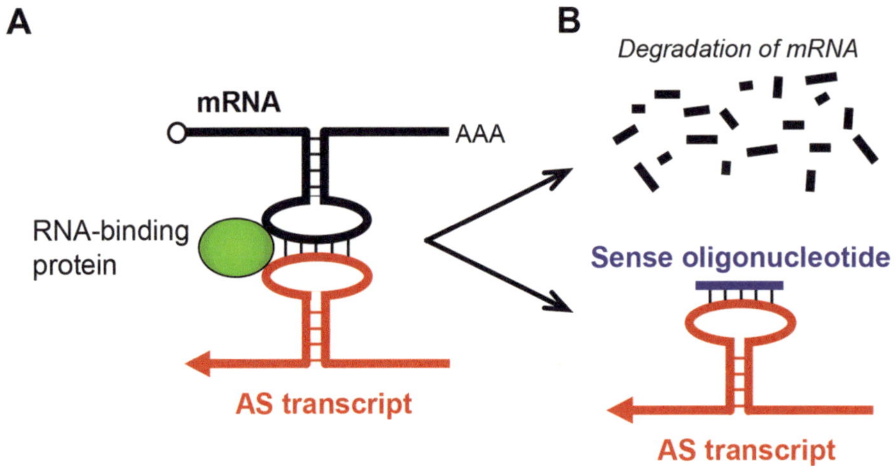

Figure 3.
A putative mechanism of the mRNA-AS transcript interaction and mRNA degradation by the introduction of a sense oligonucleotide (iNOS gene). (A) Stable complex on the iNOS mRNA. When the iNOS AS transcript is expressed, it partially hybridizes with a single-stranded loop in the iNOS mRNA that harbors a cap structure (open circle) and a poly(A) tail. By recruiting an RNA-binding protein, it forms an mRNA-AS transcript-protein complex to stabilize the iNOS mRNA in the cytoplasm. (B) Interference with the mRNA-AS transcript interaction. Because a sense oligonucleotide to the iNOS mRNA harbors the same sequence as the mRNA, it competitively inhibits the hybridization of iNOS mRNA with the iNOS AS transcript, leading to interference with the mRNA-AS transcript interaction and then the mRNA degradation. This mechanism confers to the basis of the NATRE technology.

Further analyses demonstrated that the *iNOS* AS transcript interacts with the *iNOS* mRNA at the single-stranded loop or bulge of the overlapping region between the mRNA and AS transcript (**Figure 3**) [19].

Because the orientation of RNA is 5′-to-3′, base complementarity indicates that the secondary structure of AS transcript is a mirror image of that of mRNA. This means that stem-loop structures in the AS transcript are formed at the complementary sites in the corresponding mRNA, leading to loop-loop hybridization between the mRNA and AS transcript [1, 2]. This loop-loop hybridization forms a short RNA:RNA duplex (usually <10 base pairs), which is thermodynamically unstable due to the low melting temperature of the duplex. Then, RNA-binding proteins (e.g., HuR) bind to the *iNOS* mRNA and/or AS transcript to stabilize the mRNA-AS transcript-protein complex, which protects from the degradation of RNAs and facilitates translation in the cell [19].

2.2.2 INF-A1 mRNA-AS transcript interaction

As another putative mechanism, the human *IFN-A1* AS transcript interacts with and stabilizes *IFN-A1* mRNA by blocking the microRNA binding to *IFN-A1* mRNA [20]. *IFN-A1* AS transcript is expressed at a low level. After the AS transcript transiently interacts with *IFN-A1* mRNA, it moves on and targets the next mRNA molecule in a 'hit-and-run' fashion [1, 20].

Sense oligonucleotides to BSL of *IFN-A1* mRNA (see **Figure 2**) decreased *IFN-A1* mRNA levels. Because a potent binding site of a microRNA (miR-1270) is present in BSL, miR-1270 may bind to BSL of *IFN-A1* mRNA. A microRNA-binding site is also called a microRNA-responsive element (MRE). Next, a short AS oligoribonucleotide (asORN), which is the part of *IFN-A1* AS transcript corresponding to BSL, was

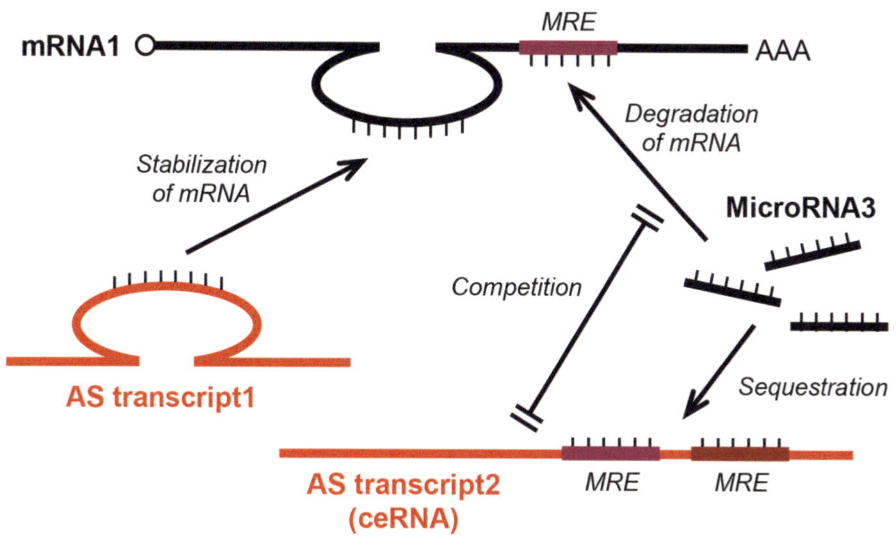

Figure 4.
A model of interactions among transcripts to regulate mRNA levels. mRNA1 has a site of interaction (loop) with AS transcript1 and an MRE for microRNA3. AS transcript1 stabilizes mRNA1, whereas microRNA destroys mRNA1 through its MRE. AS transcript2 transcribed from another gene has common MREs. AS transcript2 sponges microRNA3, resulting in the sequestration of microRNA3. Therefore, AS transcript2 competes with microRNA3 and functions as a ceRNA. A typical example is seen among IFN-A1 mRNA and AS transcripts from the specific subsets of IFN-A gene family. See details in the text.

introduced into the cells (This is not NATRE technology.). *IFN-A1* asORN increased *IFN-A1* mRNA levels, but it did not alter *IFN-A1* AS transcript levels [20]. These data imply that *IFN-A1* asORN stabilizes *IFN-A1* mRNA by simulating the AS transcript.

When the levels of transcripts were measured, miR-1270 was much more excess to *IFN-A1* AS transcript [23]. Although *IFN-A1* AS transcripts include several MREs, they are stoichiometrically unable to sponge all miR-1270 molecules. Further study indicated another mechanism.

When microRNAs are shared by mRNAs and AS transcripts, the transcripts function as competing endogenous RNAs (ceRNAs). Several AS transcripts are transcribed from the specific subsets of *IFN-A* gene family (*IFN-A1*, *A7*, *A8*, *A10*, and *A14* genes) and harbor common MREs for miR-1270 [23]. MiR-1270 can bind to both mRNA and AS transcript from *IFN-A* gene, as well as mRNAs from the specific subsets of *IFN-A* gene family (*IFN-A8*, *A10*, *A14*, and *A17* genes). Because the mRNAs and AS transcripts share MREs for miR-1270, they sponge and sequester the miR-1270 molecules. Collectively, *IFN-A* mRNAs and AS transcripts from *IFN-A* gene family form a ceRNA network to antagonize miR-1270 [23, 27]. This network finely tunes *IFN-A1* mRNA levels by common MREs that are present in the mRNAs and AS transcripts at the post-transcriptional level. Possible interactions among transcripts are depicted in **Figure 4**. See detailed discussion in [28].

2.2.3 Tnf mRNA-AS transcript interaction

Different from the *iNOS* and *IFN-A1* mRNA cases, AS transcripts sometimes downregulate gene expression. The stability of *Tnf* mRNA is modulated by RNA-binding proteins that bind to the AREs in its 3′UTR: human homolog R of embryonic lethal-abnormal visual protein (HuR), which stabilizes the mRNA; and tristetraprolin

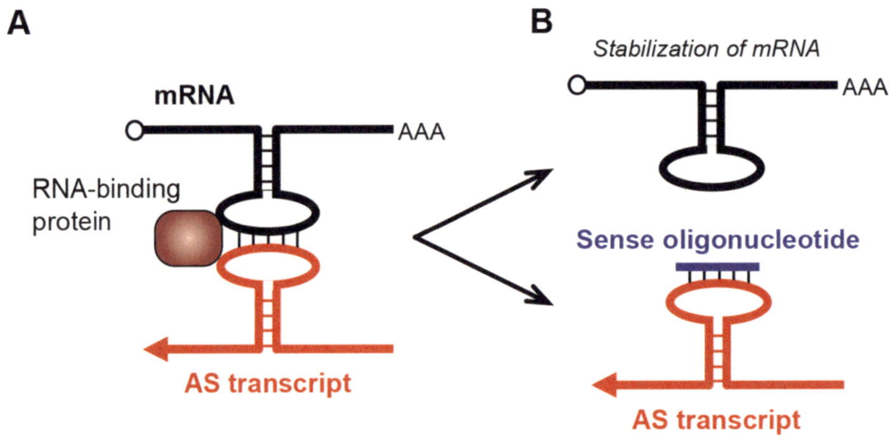

Figure 5.
A putative mechanism of the increase in mRNA levels by the introduction of a sense oligonucleotide (Tnf gene). (A) The Tnf mRNA that forms with a destabilizing RNA-binding protein. The Tnf AS transcript partially hybridizes with a single-stranded loop in the Tnf mRNA. An RNA-binding protein forms an mRNA-AS transcript-protein complex. (B) Interference with the mRNA-AS transcript interaction. A sense oligonucleotide to the Tnf mRNA competitively inhibits the hybridization of Tnf mRNA with the Tnf AS transcript, releasing a destabilizing RNA-binding protein. Finally, the Tnf mRNA becomes stable in the cytoplasm.

(TTP), which destabilizes the mRNA [24]. A putative mechanism of mRNA destabilization is schematically shown in **Figure 5** and discussed in [1, 2]. Possible involvement of microRNA in the *Tnf* mRNA-AS transcript interaction is also mentioned [24].

Other than these mechanisms, there are several AS transcript-mediated mechanisms that regulate gene expression [7]. For example, AS transcripts may epigenetically repress transcription at the chromatin level.

3. Natural antisense transcript-targeted regulation technology

3.1 Natural antisense transcript-targeted regulation technology using sense oligonucleotides

If the mRNA-AS transcript interactions are inhibited, it is speculated that an mRNA-AS transcript-protein complex is not formed and that the mRNA becomes unstable [1, 2]. According to this hypothesis, we used single-stranded *sense* oligonucleotides to block the mRNA-AS transcript interactions at a post-transcriptional level. The sense oligonucleotide harbors the same sequence as that of the relevant mRNA.

We first applied the sense oligonucleotide corresponding to the *iNOS* mRNA sequence to decrease the *iNOS* mRNA levels in hepatocytes [19]. In a search of the literature to date, there are not any other reports on applying sense oligonucleotides to knockdown AS transcript(s) and finally mRNA. After refinement of this method and confirmation of its versatility, we established this method as a natural antisense transcript-targeted regulation (NATRE) technology using sense oligonucleotides [14, 18]. The introduction of sense oligonucleotides may regulate the mRNA levels of AS transcript-expressing genes. Similarly, the sense oligonucleotides to other mRNAs reduced the levels of *IFN-A1* and other mRNAs [14, 20]. Therefore, the introduction of sense oligonucleotides may be used as loss-of-function experiments of AS transcripts.

In the absence of an AS transcript, a sense oligonucleotide cannot hybridize with the relevant mRNA and does not affect mRNA stability. Therefore, the presence of AS transcript and mRNA-AS transcript interactions are essential for the NATRE technology using sense oligonucleotides.

3.2 Design of sense oligonucleotides

3.2.1 Prediction of secondary structure

A sense oligonucleotide should harbor an overlapping sequence of an mRNA-AS transcript interaction, i.e., a single-stranded loop or bulge [18, 20]. The single-stranded loops are the potential sites of mRNA-AS transcript interactions. To seek the single-stranded regions of an mRNA where the relevant AS transcript interacts with, secondary structures of mRNA (especially, 3′UTR) were predicted using the mfold program [29]. Other prediction programs can be used. Regions conserved among predicted mRNA (especially 3′UTR) structures are selected, and candidates of several sense oligonucleotides are designed from the stem-loop regions.

Generally, it is unnecessary to predict the secondary structures of AS transcripts. As mentioned above, the overlapping sequence of an AS transcript is complementary to that of the corresponding mRNA. Therefore, the secondary structures of the AS transcript are a mirror image of the mRNA. The stems and loops of the AS transcript are formed at the same positions as the mRNA.

3.2.2 Design of sense oligonucleotides

The sense oligonucleotide consists of either synthetic oligodeoxyribonucleotide (DNA) or synthetic oligoribonucleotides (RNA) with modifications of the oligonucleotide backbone, sugars, bases, and the 5′-phosphate (described later). The sequences of sense oligonucleotides (about 20 nt long in our cases) designed according to the mRNA sequence included at least one single-stranded loop in the conserved region [14, 19]. From the sequences of sense oligonucleotides, the elements that may provoke innate immunity responses through Toll-like receptors (TLR3, 7, 8, and 9) should be eliminated, such as GU-rich motifs (e.g., 5′-GUGU-3′), CG, GGG, GGGG, and CCCC [14, 19, 30]. It is possible that some oligonucleotides show off-target effects, even after the exclusion of these motifs. To attain the specificity of a target mRNA and avoid off-target effects, homology search in the DDBJ/EMBL/GenBank databases should be performed. Trials and errors are necessary to select effective sense oligonucleotides among several candidates.

Note that not all the candidate sense oligonucleotides reduce the levels of specific mRNA species, whereas some oligonucleotides increase the mRNA levels. As abovementioned, AS transcripts modulate the expression of each gene either positively or negatively; the AS transcript stabilizes mRNA (**Figures 3** and **4**) or destabilizes mRNA (**Figure 5**).

Changes in mRNA levels also depend on the region of the mRNA-AS transcript interactions [14, 24]. Six sense oligonucleotides to the 3′UTR of the rat *Tnf* mRNA were designed to the regions whose secondary structures were conserved [24]. Among them, only one sense oligonucleotide decreased *Tnf* mRNA levels, four increased, and one did not alter. RNA-binding proteins, e.g., HuR and TTP, may change the effect of each sense oligonucleotide.

Additionally, both several RNA-binding proteins and microRNAs control the mRNA stability (see Section 2.2). Therefore, it is difficult to predict whether knockdown of AS transcript using a sense oligonucleotide causes either an increase or decrease in mRNA levels (see also Section 3.3).

3.2.3 Negative controls of sense oligonucleotides

Several types of oligonucleotides are frequently used as negative controls. A negative control that is suitable for your experiments should be selected because not all the negative controls work well in the experiments.

3.2.3.1 Sense oligonucleotides to stems

A sense oligonucleotide to stem regions is used as a negative control. A stem region consists of double-stranded RNA:RNA hybrid and is not involved in the interactions with an AS transcript [20].

3.2.3.2 Mismatch oligonucleotides or mutated oligonucleotides

Mismatch oligonucleotides are designed by introducing mutated bases at the site of mRNA-AS transcript interactions [20, 31].

3.2.3.3 Random oligonucleotides

Random oligonucleotides (20 nt) harbor random sequences, i.e., 5′-N_{20}-3′ (N = A, C, G, or T) with phosphorothioate bonds [18].

3.2.3.4 Scrambled oligonucleotides and mock transfection

A scrambled oligonucleotide is designed by base shuffling without changing the base composition of the relevant sense oligonucleotide [31]. Homology search screened by the BLAST program must eliminate candidates harboring unexpected homology to other mRNAs in the DDBJ/EMBL/GenBank databases.

When a sense oligonucleotide is introduced into cells using a transfection reagent, mock transfection is also necessary as a negative control of transfection. The mock transfection requires a transfection reagent alone, and an oligonucleotide is not introduced to the cells [18, 20].

3.2.4 Modification of sense oligonucleotides

A variety of nucleases are present in the cells and blood, such as exonuclease, endonuclease, and ribonuclease (RNase) H1. RNase activity is very high in various cell lines, as well as blood and cells in many organs, including the liver. To protect sense oligonucleotides from these nucleases, phosphorothioate bonds and modified nucleic acids are commonly introduced to replace the phosphodiester bonds and (deoxy)ribose rings of native nucleotides, respectively [32, 33]. Indeed, *iNOS* sense oligonucleotides without modification did not reduce *iNOS* mRNA levels [18]. Locked nucleic acid (LNA) [34] and 2′-*O*-methyl nucleic acid (OmeNA) are frequently used as modified nucleic acids. In our cases, *iNOS* sense oligonucleotides were substituted with partial phosphorothioate bonds and LNAs or OmeNAs reduced the levels of *iNOS* mRNA and iNOS protein in hepatocytes [18, 19]. This is a critical point at which modifications are included to obtain effective sense oligonucleotides.

3.2.5 Conjugation of sense oligonucleotides

When modified, but non-conjugated oligonucleotides are introduced in the body, they are transferred to the liver and kidney. To improve *in vivo* delivery to an organ or a tissue, sense oligonucleotides are often conjugated at their ends with cell-penetrating arginine-rich peptides and cell-permeable hydrophobic molecules [32, 33]. Cell-penetrating arginine-rich peptides are derived from the Tat protein of human immunodeficiency virus (HIV)-1 [35] and synthetic arginine oligomer peptides (Arg_6); and cell-permeable hydrophobic molecules are cholesterol [36] and C_{12} spacer.

The conjugation does not affect the potency of *iNOS* oligonucleotides to decrease *iNOS* mRNA expression [18]. When an *iNOS* sense oligonucleotide conjugated to these molecules was introduced into hepatocytes, all conjugated sense oligonucleotides were as effectively decreasing *iNOS* mRNA levels as the non-conjugated sense oligonucleotide [18]. Appropriate conjugation may facilitate the delivery of sense oligonucleotides to target tissues or organs (see Section 3.7).

3.3 Regulation of mRNA levels by sense oligonucleotides in culture cells

Because the modification of sense oligonucleotides is essential, modified sense oligonucleotides were used for the introduction to cells. The *in vitro* effects of NATRE technology (including AntagoNAT technology) on mRNA levels in the cells are summarized in **Table 1**.

mRNA levels*	Gene from which AS transcript transcribed (product)	Technology	Reference
Decrease	*iNOS* (iNOS/NOS2)	NATRE	[18, 19]
	Il23A (IL-23, alpha subunit)	NATRE	[14]
	IFN-A1 (IFN-alpha1)	NATRE	[20]
	EPHA2 (EPHA2)	NATRE	[26]
Increase	*Ccl2* (CCL2)	NATRE	[14]
	Ccl20 (CCL20)	NATRE	[14]
	Cx3xl1 (CX3CL1)	NATRE	[14]
	Cd69 (CD69)	NATRE	[14]
	RelA (NF-kappaB, p65 subunit)	NATRE	[14]
	Tnf (TNF-alpha)	NATRE	[24]
	Bdnf (BDNF)	AntagoNAT	[37]
	Gdnf (GDNF)	AntagoNAT	[37]

**Genes were classified by the main effect of sense oligonucleotides on the mRNA levels.*

Table 1.
Examples of the in vitro effects of NATRE technology on mRNA levels.

3.4 Administration of sense oligonucleotides to animals

When NO is excessively produced by iNOS in hepatocytes and Kupffer cells (resident macrophages) of the liver, it leads to multiple organ failure [38]. Endotoxemia model rats with hepatic failure are often used to evaluate drugs. These model rats are prepared either by intravenous injection of D-galactosamine (GalN) and LPS [38–40], or by LPS injection after partial hepatectomy [38, 41]. These rats resemble the animals suffering from sepsis or septic shock.

After optimization of the sequence and modification of *iNOS* sense oligonucleotides in hepatocytes, the best sense oligonucleotide was administered into the endotoxemia model rats [38]. When the sense oligonucleotide was intravenously injected with GalN and LPS to rats, the survival rate was markedly increased, and apoptosis in the hepatocytes markedly decreased in the sense oligonucleotide-treated rats [38].

Because LNA is efficiently accumulated in the liver [34], the LNA-modified *iNOS* sense oligonucleotide may function in the liver where the *iNOS* gene is highly expressed. Taken together, NATRE technology using *iNOS* sense oligonucleotides may be applicable to treat sepsis and septic shock.

3.5 AntagoNAT technology

To increase mRNA levels by modulating the mRNA-AS transcript interactions, an *AntagoNAT* oligonucleotide has been used, which is an antagonist to an AS transcript (NAT) and defined as a single-stranded antisense oligonucleotide to a specific AS transcript [37]. Each AntagoNAT oligonucleotide contained a mixture of OmeNAs and LNAs.

When an AS transcript overlaps with its corresponding mRNA, the AntagoNAT is identical to a sense oligonucleotide. Therefore, AntagoNAT technique is very close to NATRE technology. Both technologies use sense oligonucleotides to knockdown AS transcript. However, NATRE technology has been applied to decrease mRNA levels, whereas AntagoNAT technology has been applied to increase mRNA levels.

It has been reported that AntagoNAT-mediated knockdown of brain-derived neurotrophic factor (*Bdnf*) and glial-derived neurotrophic factor (*Gdnf*) AS transcripts resulted in increased levels of *Bdnf* and *Gdnf* mRNAs in HEK293T cells [37]. The underlying mechanism may be similar to those indicated in **Figure 5**, or to other mechanisms that were previously mentioned [7].

AntagoNAT oligonucleotides can be administered to animals. When *Bdnf*-AntagoNAT was intracerebroventricularly delivered, the *Bdnf* mRNA levels increased in the mouse brain [37]. Collectively, the *Bdnf*-AntagoNATs functioned *in vitro* and *in vivo*, although it increased the *Bdnf* mRNA levels.

AntagomiR (antagomir), which is a synthetic oligonucleotide complementary to a microRNA, is used to sequester endogenous microRNA [42]. Each antagomir sequence is identical to a specific mRNA and similar to several mRNAs that share microRNA-binding sites (seed sequences). Therefore, antagomirs are another type of sense oligonucleotides. When microRNA is involved in the mRNA-AS transcript interactions, the antagomir technology may be applied to analyze these interactions. See an example in [23].

3.6 Comparison with other methods

The mechanisms of two conventional technologies, i.e., antisense and siRNA technologies [11], are schematically shown (**Figure 6**).

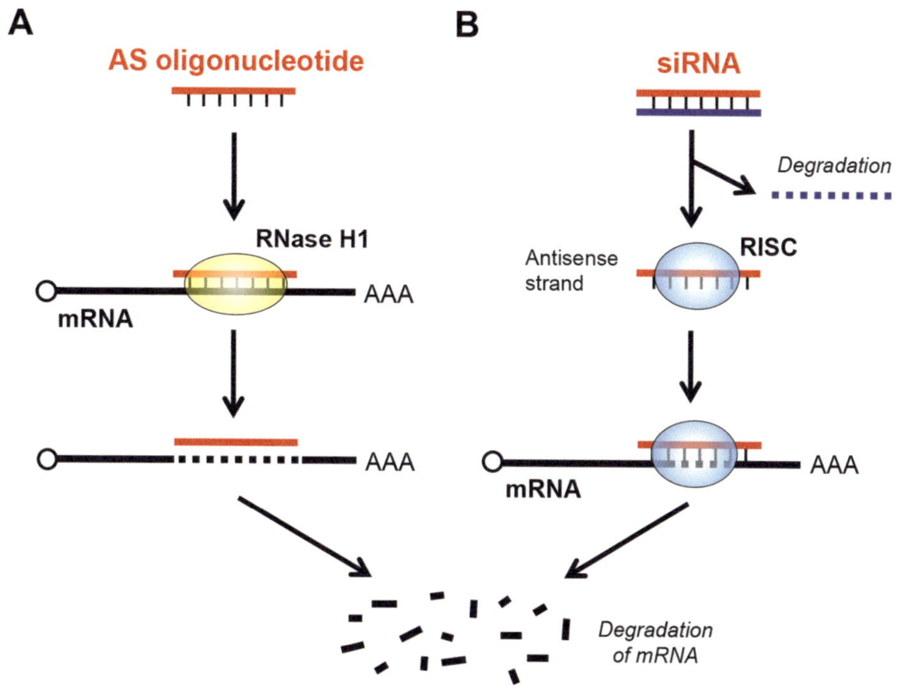

Figure 6.
Mechanisms of conventional mRNA knockdown technologies. (A) Antisense technology. The mRNA that hybridizes with an antisense oligonucleotide is digested by RNase H1. (B) siRNA technology. siRNA recruits Argonaut (Ago) proteins to form RISC, which destroys mRNA. See details in the text.

3.6.1 Antisense technology

A single-stranded antisense oligonucleotide hybridizes with an mRNA and forms a local DNA:RNA hybrid. RNase H1 recognizes DNA:RNA hybrids and selectively digests the RNA strand, leading to the degradation of the mRNA. Therefore, the antisense oligonucleotides should be DNA. The presence of an AS transcript is not essential for this method.

3.6.2 siRNA technology

siRNA is a synthetic double-stranded RNA, and one strand of the siRNA (i.e., guide strand) is complementary to a target mRNA. Typical siRNA consists of 19 base pairs and 2-nt 3′ overhangs. siRNA interacts with Argonaut (Ago) proteins to form RNA-induced silencing complex (RISC) and then binds to the target mRNA. The guide strand of siRNA hybridizes with the mRNA (especially, 3′UTR) in the RISC, resulting in degradation of the target mRNA. The other RNA strand (i.e., passenger strand) is destroyed during the RISC formation. This mechanism mimics mRNA degradation by microRNA.

As mRNA knockdown methods, NATRE technology using sense oligonucleotides is compared with conventional methods, i.e., antisense technology and siRNA technology (**Table 2**). Other than these technologies, there are various oligonucleotide technologies that are applied to therapies of disease.

	NATRE technology	Antisense technology	siRNA technology
Targets	AS transcript (direct) and mRNA (indirect)	mRNAs	mRNAs
Oligonucleotides* (strand)	Single-stranded DNA or RNA (sense)	Single-stranded DNA (antisense)	Double-stranded RNA (both)
Underlying mechanism	mRNA-AS transcript interactions**	None	None
mRNA degradation	RNases and other nucleases	RNase H1	RISC
Disadvantage	Impossible when mRNA-AS transcript interactions are absent	Difficult to optimize the sequence to the relevant mRNA	Difficult when stable secondary structures are present
Examples of human application	Not yet (Successful results in animal experiments)	Mipomersen, casimersen, etc. [11]	Patisiran, givosiran, etc. [11]

**The backbone, sugars, bases, and the 5′-phosphate of the oligonucleotide are modified.*
***MicroRNAs may interfere with these interactions.*

Table 2.
Comparison of the methods to knockdown mRNAs.

3.6.3 RNA aptamers

Aptamers are oligoribonucleotides that form 3D structures and function like proteins, such as ligands and antibodies [42]. For example, pegaptanib, which is an aptamer drug developed for the treatment of macular degeneration, blocks vascular endothelial growth factor (VEGF) by preventing its binding to VEGF receptors [42]. Although there are no reports about the mRNA knockdown using aptamers up to date, the aptamers that simulate RNA-binding proteins may be utilized to modulate mRNA levels by affecting the mRNA-AS transcript interactions.

3.7 Drug delivery system (DDS)

The introduction of oligonucleotides to cells requires transfection reagents using liposomes, e.g., Lipofectamine (Thermo Fisher Scientific Inc., Waltham, MA, USA) and using iron nanoparticles, e.g., MATra A reagent (IBA, Göttingen, Germany) or PolyMag Magnetofection reagent (OZ Biosciences, Marseille, France).

To improve the *in vivo* delivery of sense oligonucleotides, several techniques have been developed [32, 33]. Because LNA is efficiently accumulated in the liver [34], *iNOS* sense oligonucleotides were modified with LNAs [38].

Recently, *N*-acetylgalactosamine (GalNAc) has been conjugated at the ends of the oligonucleotides to efficiently deliver the oligonucleotides to the liver [11, 43]. Because the liver and kidney receive high blood flow and permeability of their capillaries is high, sense oligonucleotides conjugated with GalNAc will improve the delivery and accumulation in these organs. To cross the blood-brain barrier, *Bdnf*-AntagoNATs in liposomes were delivered by nasal approaches [44, 45]. Additionally, aptamers capable of entering the cells may facilitate the delivery of oligonucleotides into the cells [42].

Because guinea pigs maintain a functional *MX1* gene for the IFN-alpha1 pathway, they were infected with influenza virus to verify that the AS transcript-mRNA regulatory axis exerts *in vivo* control of innate immunity [46]. When an AS oligoribonucleotide (asORN) to guinea pig *IFN-A1* mRNA in poly (D,L-lactide-co-glycolide (PLGA) nanoparticles was pulmonary-administered, it inhibited *in vivo* viral proliferation by modulating *IFN-A1* mRNA levels. Although this experiment is not NATRE technology, PLGA nanoparticles can be used to deliver sense oligonucleotides to animals. Various lipid nanoparticles (LNPs) have been used to deliver nucleic acids, including oligonucleotides, in the body [47]. New-generation LNPs can deliver long RNA, such as LNP-based mRNA vaccines for COVID-19 [47].

4. Perspectives

Administration of oligonucleotides, including NATRE technology, is a unique therapeutic modality. Because the sequence of an oligonucleotide specifies the gene, one mRNA is selectively downregulated or upregulated (**Figure 7**). For example, administration of an *iNOS* sense oligonucleotide to endotoxemia/sepsis model rats showed little effects on endothelial NOS (eNOS) and neuronal NOS (nNOS) (unpublished data). Enzyme inhibitors (e.g., NOS inhibitors) generally have a broader specificity. Furthermore, it is rare that antibodies against oligonucleotides are raised.

NATRE technology is a powerful method to modulate *in vitro* and *in vivo* gene expression. Note that sense oligonucleotides to the mRNAs can be designed to inducible genes and many other genes. iNOS AS transcript was successfully administered to endotoxemia/sepsis model rats and improved their survival rate [38]. As shown in **Table 1**, many genes involved in inflammation are candidates suitable for clinical uses in the future. When a gene that is involved in diseases is selected, sense oligonucleotides to this gene can be easily designed and examined. Instead of sense oligonucleotides, antisense oligoribonucleotides (asORN) may be used to increase mRNA levels. Indeed, *IFN-A1* asORN inhibited the proliferation of Influenza virus in guinea pigs [46].

Sense oligonucleotides may apply to cancer, neurodegenerative disorders, and other diseases. For example, EPHA2 is over-expressed in various cancers, and the *EPHA2*

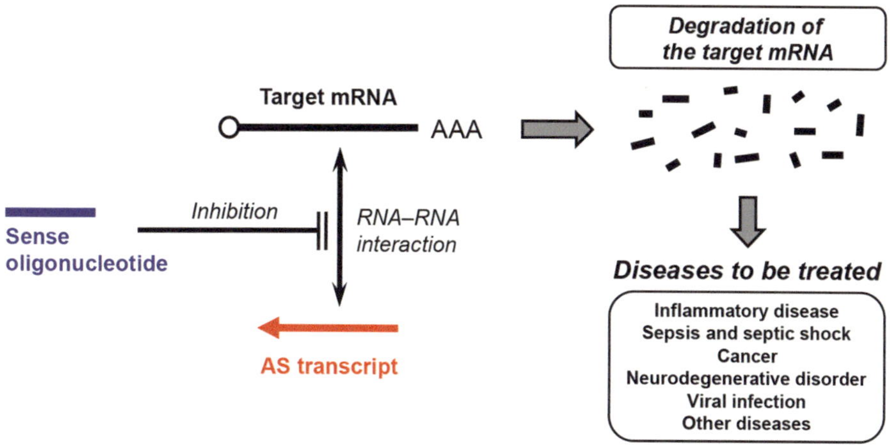

Figure 7.
The NATRE technology using sense oligonucleotides. The principle of the NATRE technology is schematically shown. Potential therapeutic application using this technology is also shown.

AS transcript may be involved in a subtype of breast cancer [26]. It is possible that sense oligonucleotides inhibit cancer progression and proliferation of cancer cells. Furthermore, the administration of *Bdnf*- and *Gdnf*-AntagoNATs to mice [44, 45] may facilitate the regeneration of neurons and glial cells in the central nervous system. When a gene that is involved in diseases is found, sense oligonucleotides to this gene can be designed. Furthermore, sense oligonucleotides can be designed in the genome of a pathogenic virus to inhibit viral multiplication.

Drugs and some constituents in functional foods and crude drugs of Japanese Kampo medicine mimic sense oligonucleotides by modulating mRNA stability [1]. When sodium salicylate reduced *iNOS* mRNA levels in hepatocytes, decreased mRNA stability was speculated [48]. It was reported that acetyl salicylate (aspirin) interacts with RNA by intercalating with the RNA duplex and destabilized the helix, resulting in a conformational change of the stem-loop structure of the RNA [49]. Because the drug-RNA interaction may affect mRNA stability, drugs and constituents may interfere with *iNOS* mRNA-AS transcript interactions like sense oligonucleotides. Indeed, several drugs or constituents in functional foods and crude drugs decreased the levels of both *iNOS* mRNA and AS transcript: dexamethasone (anti-inflammatory drug) [50], cucurbitacin B (triterpenoid in the fruit of *Momordica charantia*) [51], sakuranetin (flavonoid in the bark of *Prunus jamasakura*) [52], and standardized oligomerized-polyphenol from *Litchi chinensis* fruit extract (OPLFE) [53]. The investigation of the drugs and constituents may clarify the mechanism of action of the sense oligonucleotide in future.

5. Conclusion

When AS transcript is transcribed from a gene, NATRE technology can be applied to any gene to down- or up-regulate mRNA levels. NATRE technology using sense oligonucleotides may be useful to specifically inhibit mRNA-AS transcript interactions. Therefore, this method may be applied to many genes and contribute to the treatment of various human diseases in the future.

Acknowledgements

We thank Drs. Tominori Kimura, Tadayoshi Okumura, and Saki Shirako (Ritsumeikan University) for their valuable advice and discussion and Ms. Noriko Kanazawa for her secretarial assistance. This work was supported in part by the Japan Society for the Promotion of Science KAKENHI Grant Nos. 21K08697, 21K09032, and 19KK0413 and by the Asia-Japan Research Institute, Ritsumeikan University (Ibaraki, Osaka, Japan).

Conflict of interest

M.N. is an inventor of a patent describing the use of *iNOS* sense oligonucleotides to regulate *iNOS* mRNA levels. The other authors declare no conflict of interest.

Author details

Mikio Nishizawa[1]*, Tetsuya Okuyama[2] and Richi Nakatake[2]

1 Department of Biomedical Sciences, College of Life Sciences, Ritsumeikan University, Kusatsu, Shiga, Japan

2 Department of Surgery, Kansai Medical University, Hirakata, Osaka, Japan

*Address all correspondence to: nishizaw@sk.ritsumei.ac.jp

References

[1] Nishizawa M, Okumura T, Ikeya Y, Kimura T. Regulation of inducible gene expression by natural antisense transcripts. Frontiers in Bioscience (Landmark Ed.). 2012;**17**:938-958. DOI: 10.2741/3965

[2] Nishizawa M, Ikeya Y, Okumura T, Kimura T. Post-transcriptional inducible gene regulation by natural antisense RNA. Frontiers in Bioscience (Landmark Ed.). 2015;**20**:1-36. DOI: 10.2741/4297

[3] Kiyosawa H, Mise N, Iwase S, Hayashizaki Y, Abe K. Disclosing hidden transcripts: Mouse natural sense-antisense transcripts tend to be poly(A) negative and nuclear localized. Genome Research. 2005;**15**:463-474. DOI: 10.1101/gr.3155905

[4] Wright MW. A short guide to long non-coding RNA gene nomenclature. Human Genomics. 2014;**8**:7. DOI: 10.1186/1479-7364-8-7

[5] Lee RC, Feinbaum RL, Ambros V. The *C. elegans* heterochronic gene lin-4 encodes small RNAs with antisense complementarity to lin-14. Cell. 1993;**75**:843-854. DOI: 10.1016/0092-8674(93)90529-y

[6] Wilusz JE, Sunwoo H, Spector DL. Long noncoding RNAs: Functional surprises from the RNA world. Genes & Development. 2009;**23**:1494-1504. DOI: 10.1101/gad.1800909

[7] Faghihi MA, Wahlestedt C. Regulatory roles of natural antisense transcripts. Nature Reviews Molecular Cell Biology. 2009;**10**:637-643. DOI: 10.1038/nrm2738

[8] Volders PJ, Anckaert J, Verheggen K, Nuytens J, Martens L, Mestdagh P, et al. LNCipedia 5: Towards a reference set of human long non-coding RNAs. Nucleic Acids Research. 2019;**47**:D135-D139. DOI: 10.1093/nar/gky1031

[9] Morris KV, Mattick JS. The rise of regulatory RNA. Nature Reviews Genetics. 2014;**15**:423-437. DOI: 10.1038/nrg3722

[10] Krappinger JC, Bonstingl L, Pansy K, Sallinger K, Wreglesworth NI, Grinninger L, et al. Non-coding natural antisense transcripts: Analysis and application. Journal of Biotechnology. 2021;**340**:75-101. DOI: 10.1016/j.jbiotec.2021.08.005

[11] Crook S, Liang XH, Baker BF, Crook RM. Antisense technology: A review. Journal of Biological Chemistry. 2021;**296**:100416. DOI: 10.1016/j.jbc.2021.100416

[12] Dykxhoorn DM, Lieberman J. The silent revolution: RNA interference as basic biology, research tool, and therapeutic. Annual Review of Medicine. 2005;**56**:401-423. DOI: 10.1146/annurev.med.56.082103.104606

[13] Wahlestedt C. Natural antisense and noncoding RNA transcripts as potential drug targets. Drug Discovery Today. 2006;**11**:503-508. DOI: 10.1016/j.drudis.2006.04.013

[14] Yoshigai E, Hara T, Okuyama T, Okumura T, Kaibori M, Kwon AH, et al. Characterization of natural antisense transcripts expressed from interleukin 1beta-inducible genes in rat hepatocytes. HOAJ Biology. 2012;**1**:10. DOI: 10.7243/2050-0874-1-10

[15] Jing Q, Huang S, Guth S, Zarubin T, Motoyama A, Chen, et al. Involvement of

microRNA in AU-rich element-mediated mRNA instability. Cell. 2005;**120**:623-634. DOI: 10.1016/j.cell.2004.12.038

[16] Hogan DJ, Riordan DP, Gerber AP, Herschlag D, Brown PO. Diverse RNA-binding proteins interact with functionally related sets of RNAs, suggesting an extensive regulatory system. PLoS Biology. 2008;**6**:e255. DOI: 10.1371/journal.pbio.0060255

[17] Yoshida H, Kwon AH, Habara K, Yamada M, Kaibori M, Kamiyama Y, et al. Edaravone inhibits the induction of iNOS gene expression at transcriptional and posttranscriptional steps in murine macrophages. Shock. 2008;**30**:734-739. DOI: 10.1097/SHK.0b013e318173ea0b

[18] Yoshigai E, Hara T, Araki Y, Tanaka Y, Oishi M, Tokuhara K, et al. Natural antisense transcript-targeted regulation of inducible nitric oxide synthase mRNA levels. Nitric Oxide. 2013;**30**:9-16. DOI: 10.1016/j.niox.2013.01.001

[19] Matsui K, Nishizawa M, Ozaki T, Kimura T, Hashimoto I, Yamada M, et al. Natural antisense transcript stabilizes inducible nitric oxide synthase messenger RNA in rat hepatocytes. Hepatology. 2008;**47**:686-697. DOI: 10.1002/hep.22036

[20] Kimura T, Jiang S, Nishizawa M, Yoshigai E, Hashimoto I, Nishikawa M, et al. Stabilization of human interferon-alpha1 mRNA by its antisense RNA. Cellular and Molecular Life Sciences. 2013;**70**:1451-1467. DOI: 10.1007/s00018-012-1216-x

[21] Kimura T, Hashimoto I, Nishizawa M, Ito S, Yamada H. Novel cis-active structures in the coding region mediate CRM1-dependent nuclear export of IFN-alpha1 mRNA. Medical Molecular Morphology. 2010;**43**:145-157. DOI: 10.1007/s00795-010-0492-5

[22] Génin P, Vaccaro A, Civas A. The role of differential expression of human interferon—A genes in antiviral immunity. Cytokine & Growth Factor Reviews. 2009;**20**:283-295. DOI: 10.1016/j.cytogfr.2009.07.005

[23] Kimura T, Jiang S, Yoshida N, Sakamoto R, Nishizawa M. Interferon-alpha1 competing endogenous RNA network antagonizes microRNA-1270. Cellular and Molecular Life Sciences. 2015;**72**:2749-2761. DOI: 10.1007/s00018-015-1875-5

[24] Yoshigai E, Hara T, Inaba H, Hashimoto I, Tanaka Y, Kaibori M, et al. Interleukin-1beta induces tumor necrosis factor-alpha secretion from rat hepatocytes. Hepatology Research. 2014;**44**:571-583. DOI: 10.1111/hepr.12157

[25] Sakamoto R, Kumagai K, Odaka T, Okuyama T, Nishizawa M, Kimura T. A standardized suppresses breast cancer cell proliferation by regulating the expression of EphA2 antisense RNA–mRNA axis independently of microRNA. Bioactive Compounds in Health and Disease. 2019;**2**:191-205. DOI: 10.31989/bchd.v2i9.642

[26] Okuyama T, Sakamoto R, Kumagai K, Nishizawa M, Kimura T, Sugie T, et al. EPHA2 antisense RNA modulates EPHA2 mRNA levels in basal-like/triple-negative breast cancer cells. Biochimie. 2020;**179**:169-180. DOI: 10.1016/j.biochi.2020.10.002

[27] Nishizawa M, Kimura T. RNA networks that regulate mRNA expression and their potential as drug targets. RNA & DISEASE. 2016;**3**:e864. DOI: 10.14800/rd.864

[28] Kimura T. Non-coding natural antisense RNA: Mechanisms of action in the regulation of target gene expression

and its clinical implications. Yakugaku Zasshi. 2020;**140**:687-700. DOI: 10.1248/yakushi.20-00002

[29] Zuker M. Mfold web server for nucleic acid folding and hybridization prediction. Nucleic Acids Research. 2003;**31**:3406-3415. DOI: 10.1093/nar/gkg595

[30] Forsbach A, Nemorin JG, Montino C, Muller C, Samulowitz U, Vicari AP, et al. Identification of RNA sequence motifs stimulating sequence-specific TLR8-dependent immune responses. Journal of Immunology. 2008;**180**:3729-3738. DOI: 10.4049/jimmunol.180.6.3729

[31] Muratani T, Nishizawa M, Matsumura S, Mabuchi T, Abe K, Shimamoto K, et al. Functional characterization of prostaglandin F2alpha receptor in the spinal cord for tactile pain (allodynia). Journal of Neurochemistry. 2003;**86**:374-382. DOI: 10.1046/j.1471-4159.2003.01840.x

[32] Khvorova A, Watts JK. The chemical evolution of oligonucleotide therapies of clinical utility. Nature Biotechnology. 2017;**35**:238-248. DOI: 10.1038/nbt.3765

[33] Johannes L, Lucchino M. Current challenges in delivery and cytosolic translocation of therapeutic RNAs. Nucleic Acid Therapeutics. 2018;**28**:178-193. DOI: 10.1089/nat.2017.0716

[34] Straarup EM, Fisker N, Hedtjärn M, Lindholm MW, Rosenbohm C, Aarup V, et al. Short locked nucleic acid antisense oligonucleotides potently reduce apolipoprotein B mRNA and serum cholesterol in mice and non-human primates. Nucleic Acids Research. 2010;**38**:7100-7111. DOI: 10.1093/nar/gkq457

[35] Abes S, Moulton H, Turne J, Clair P, Richard JP, Iversen P, et al. Peptide-based delivery of nucleic acids: Design, mechanism of uptake and applications to splice-correcting oligonucleotides. Biochemical Society Transactions. 2007;**35**:53-55. DOI: 10.1042/BST0350053

[36] Holasová S, Mojzísek M, Buncek M, Vokurková D, Radilová H, Safárová M, et al. Cholesterol conjugated oligonucleotide and LNA: A comparison of cellular and nuclear uptake by Hep2 cells enhanced by Streptolysin-O. Molecular and Cellular Biochemistry. 2005;**276**:61-69. DOI: 10.1007/s11010-005-2912-8

[37] Modarresi F, Faghihi MA, Lopez-Toledano MA, Fatemi RP, Magistri M, Brothers SP, et al. Inhibition of natural antisense transcripts in vivo results in gene-specific transcriptional upregulation. Nature Biotechnology. 2012;**30**:453-459. DOI: 10.1038/nbt.2158

[38] Okuyama T, Nakatake R, Kaibori M, Okumura T, Kon M, Nishizawa M. A sense oligonucleotide to inducible nitric oxide synthase mRNA increases the survival rate of rats in septic shock. Nitric Oxide. 2018;**72**:32-40. DOI: 10.1016/j.niox.2017.11.003

[39] Tanaka H, Uchida Y, Kaibori M, Hijikawa T, Ishizaki M, Yamada M, et al. Na^+/H^+ exchanger inhibitor, FR183998, has protective effect in lethal acute liver failure and prevents iNOS induction in rats. Journal of Hepatology. 2008;**48**:289-299. DOI: 10.1016/j.jhep.2007.09.017

[40] Hijikawa T, Kaibori M, Uchida Y, Yamada M, Matsui K, Ozaki T, et al. Insulin-like growth factor 1 prevents liver injury through the inhibition of TNF-alpha and iNOS induction in D-galactosamine and LPS-treated rats. Shock. 2008;**29**:740-747. DOI: 10.1097/SHK.0b013e31815d0780

[41] Nakatake R, Tanaka Y, Ueyama Y, Miki H, Ishizaki M, Matsui K, et al.

Protective effects of active hexose correlated compound in a rat model of liver injury after hepatectomy. Functional Foods in Health and Disease. 2016;**6**:702-717. DOI: 10.31989/ffhd.v6i11.305

[42] Lundin KE, Gissberg O, Smith CIE. Oligonucleotide therapies: The past and the present. Human Gene Therapy. 2015;**26**:475-485. DOI: 10.1089/hum.2015.070

[43] Debacker AJ, Voutila J, Catley M, Blakey D, Habib N. Delivery of oligonucleotides to the liver with GalNAc: From research to registered therapeutic drug. Molecular Therapy. 2020;**28**:1759-1771. DOI: 10.1016/j.ymthe.2020.06.015

[44] Padmakumar S, Jones G, Khorkova O, Hsiao J, Kim J, Bleier BS, et al. Osmotic core-shell polymeric implant for sustained BDNF AntagoNAT delivery in CNS using minimally invasive nasal depot (MIND) approach. Biomaterials. 2021;**276**:120989. DOI: 10.1016/j.biomaterials.2021.120989

[45] Pawar G, Parayath NN, Sharma AA, Coito C, Khorkova O, Hsiao J, et al. Endonasal CNS delivery system for blood-brain barrier Impermeant therapeutic oligonucleotides using heterotopic mucosal engrafting. Frontiers in Pharmacology. 2021;**12**:660841. DOI: 10.3389/fphar.2021.660841

[46] Sakamoto R, Jiang S, Tsukada Y, Tsujimoto H, Kimura T. IFN-Alpha1 antisense RNA represses human influenza A virus growth in a Guinea pig system. Frontiers in Bioscience (Landmark Ed.). 2019;**24**:798-818. DOI: 10.2741/4752

[47] Tenchov R, Bird R, Curtze AE, Zhou Q. Lipid nanoparticles—From liposomes to mRNA vaccine delivery, a landscape of research diversity and advancement. ACS Nano. 2021;**15**:16982-17015. DOI: 10.1021/acsnano.1c04996

[48] Sakitani K, Kitade H, Lnoue K, Kamiyama Y, Nishizawa M, Okumura T, et al. The anti-inflammatory drug sodium salicylate inhibits nitric oxide formation induced by interleukin-1beta at a translational step, but not at a transcriptional step, in hepatocytes. Hepatology. 1997;**25**:416-420. DOI: 10.1053/jhep.1997.v25.pm0009021956

[49] Neault JF, Tajmir-Riahi HA. RNA-aspirin interaction studied by FTIR difference spectroscopy. Journal of Physical Chemistry B. 1997;**101**:114-116. DOI: 10.1021/jp9619292

[50] Ozaki T, Habara K, Matsui K, Kaibori M, Kwon AH, Ito S, et al. Dexamethasone inhibits the induction or iNOS gene expression through destabilization of its mRNA in proinflammatory cytokine-stimulated hepatocytes. Shock. 2010;**33**:64-69. DOI: 10.1097/SHK.0b013e3181a7fd74

[51] Dwijayanti DR, Okuyama T, Okumura T, Ikeya Y, Nishizawa M. The anti-inflammatory effects of Indonesian and Japanese bitter melon (*Momordica charantia* L.) fruit extracts on interleukin-1beta-treated hepatocytes. Functional Foods in Health and Disease. 2019;**9**:16-33. DOI: 10.31989/ffhd.v9i1.560

[52] Yamauchi Y, Okuyama T, Ishii T, Okumura T, Ikeya Y, Nishizawa M. Sakuranetin downregulates inducible nitric oxide synthase expression by affecting interleukin-1 receptor and CCAAT/enhancer-binding protein beta. Journal of Natural Medicines. 2019;**73**:353-368. DOI: 10.1007/s11418-018-1267-x

[53] Yamanishi R, Yoshigai E, Okuyama T, Mori M, Murase H, Machida T, et al. The anti-inflammatory effects of Flavanol-rich lychee fruit extract in rat hepatocytes. PLoS One. 2014;**9**:e93818. DOI: 10.1371/journal.pone.0093818

Chapter 6

Identification of RNA Oligonucleotide and Protein Interactions Using Term Frequency Inverse Document Frequency and Random Forest

Eugene Uwiragiye and Kristen L. Rhinehardt

Abstract

The interaction between protein and Ribonucleic Acid (RNA) plays crucial roles in many biological aspects such as gene expression, posttranscriptional regulation, and protein synthesis. However, the experimental screening of protein-RNA binding affinity is laborious and time-consuming, there is a pressing desire of accurate and reliable computational approaches. In this study, we proposed a novel method to predict that interaction based on both sequences of protein and RNA. The Random Forest was trained and tested on a combination of benchmark datasets and the term frequency–inverse document frequency method combined with XgBoost algorithm was used to extract useful information from sequences. The performance of our method was very impressive, and the accuracy was as high as 94%, the Area Under the Curve of 0.98 and the Matthew Correlation Coefficient (MCC) of 0.90. All these high metrics, especially the MCC, show that our method is robust enough to keep its performance on unseen datasets.

Keywords: protein, RNA, interaction, random forest, TFIDF, machine learning

1. Introduction

The protein-RNA pairs are highly involved in various regulatory processes. Finding the binding sites of the RNA-binding Proteins (RBP) is therefore an important research goal. Studies have shown that RBPs bind to RNA molecules by recognizing both sequences (sequence motifs) and secondary structure contexts (structure motifs) [1–4]. Some of them have been based on sequence-derived features such as amino acid composition, dipeptide composition, composition-transition-distribution of seven physicochemical properties, evolutionary information in terms of position-specific scoring matrices and functional domain composition [5–7]. Although progress has been made in the implementation of predictive methods for RBPs, insufficient attention has been paid to the development of predictive methods for RNA-protein

IntechOpen

interactions (RPI). The history is brief, and there are not many existing computational tools because of the scarcity of available data [8].

The machine learning (ML) methods, which have become standard tools in many fields of science and engineering, are computationally efficient methods that employs computer science, artificial intelligence, computational statistics, and information theory to fit high-dimensional models to large amounts of data. The ML methods read in data points which are generated within some application domain and each data point is characterized by two properties, such as features (predictor variables) and labels (predicted variables). The machine learning algorithms aims at learning to predict the label of a data point based solely on the features of this data point or identify the pattern those data points if they are neither classified nor labeled. The ML algorithms applied to labeled data points is called supervised learning in contrast to unsupervised learning which does not require knowing the label value of any data point. The dataset we used in this research was tagged with known labels (binding pairs are labeled as positive while non-binding pairs are labeled as negative). While the principle behind supervised ML sounds trivial, the challenge of modern ML applications is the data points non-linearity and complexity. This research focuses on three supervised learning algorithms: Logistic Regression, Random Forest, and Multinomial Naïve Bayesian.

The logistic regression is a binary classification method that can be applied to data points with feature vector $X \in R^n$ and binary labels y. These binary labels take on values from a label space that contains two different label values (most cases y = {0,1}). The linear operator $h(x) = w^T x$, with $w \in R^n$, can take an arbitrary real random number and can predict the label y when compared to a given threshold. The data point with feature x would be classified as y = 1 if the $h\ (x) \geq 0$ and $y = 0$ *if the* $h(x) < 0$. The multinomial naïve Bayesian is a simple but important probabilistic model which is defined by a function h from the feature space X to the label space Y ($h : X \rightarrow Y$) such that the predicted value $h(x), x \in X$, agrees enough with the true value $y \in Y$. The random forest is a flowchart-like description of a function from the feature space to label space that maps the features to their respective labels. While a random forest can be applied to an arbitrary feature space, we will discuss it for a specific space later in this paper.

In 2011, Pancaldi and Bähler [8–10] predicted the RNA-binding proteins and messanger-RNA using two conventional machine learning classifiers: support vector machine (SVM) and random forest (RF), while Bellucci et al. developed an algorithm called catRAPID to facilitate the predictions of 592 RPIs from the Protein Database Bank (PDB). They used the physicochemical properties of sequences as features and found three most predictive features: secondary structure propensities, hydrogen bonding, and van der Waals [8, 11]. The two benchmark datasets, called RPI369 and RPI2241, were constructed from PRIDB (a database of protein-RNA interfaces) [8, 12, 13] and achieved remarkable prediction accuracies on these two datasets using Conjoint Triad Feature (CTF) and normalized 4-gram frequencies. In 2013, the CatRAPID Omics was generated as an improved CatRAPID that used the information on protein and RNA domains involved in macromolecular recognition [8, 14, 15]. Zhao Hui-Zhan et al. [8, 16] proposed a deep learning model to predict RPIs using bi-gram from Position Specific Scoring Matrix (PSSM) approaches to extract features from proteins, and k-mers approach combined with a stacked auto-encoder for RNAs feature extraction.

In 2015, Suresh et al. [8, 17] integrated sequence information and predicted structure together to produce an accurate prediction of non-coding RNA-protein pairs on a newly constructed dataset, called RPI1807. When tested on the RPI369 and RPI2241 datasets mentioned above, some improvements were achieved on prediction accuracies. In 2017, Liu et al. proposed a semi-supervised method called LPI-NRLMF [18, 19] to predict lncRNA-protein interactions by neighborhood regularized logistic matrix factorization. One year later, Zhao et al. came up with IRWNRLPI method [20], integrating random walk and neighborhood regularized logistic matrix factorization for lncRNA-protein interactions prediction and LPI-BNPRA method using the bipartite network projection recommended algorithm to identify lncRNA-protein interactions. The last four semi-supervised methods and the BNPMDA method proposed by Chen et al. [21] in late 2018, performed well only on interactive pairs with a high predictive accuracy but weakly for non-interactive pairs. In 2018, Hu et al. proposed HLPI Ensemble method [22] for identifying lncRNA-protein interactions in human only, which integrated three common machine learning algorithms, SVM, RF and Extreme Gradient Boosting (XGB).

All the machine learning methods discussed above, use handcrafted features from proteins. In this study we proposed a new method, called TF-IDF borrowed from natural language processing, to extract features from RPI pairs. The TF-IDF standing for Term Frequency–Inverse Document Frequency takes as input a sequence of strings and transform it into a vector of numerical values.

2. Material and methodology

According to Hongchu Wang and Pengfei Wu in 2017 [8] there are 1973 RPI complexes available in the Protein Data Bank (PDB), which contains over 15,000 protein chains and more than 3000 RNA chains. However, according to research using high-throughput sequencing techniques (such as RNA-Seq), at least 30,000 lncRNAs were identified by 2013. In this study we combined the three different datasets; The RPI2241 dataset, containing 2241 RNA–protein pairs was extracted from PRIDB [13] and reconstructed by Wang in 2013, the RPI488, a non-redundant lncRPI dataset based on structural complexes which consists of 488 lncRNA-protein pairs, including 245 non-interacting pairs and 243 interacting pairs from Pan et al. [23, 24] and the RPI12737 dataset containing 12,737 experimentally validated RNA–protein pairs that extracted from NPInter v2.0 database [25]. This dataset contains the same number of non-interacting RNA–protein pairs (negative examples) as the number of interacting RNA–protein pairs. After the dataset combination, we cleaned the data by removing all pairs containing a non-amino acid character for proteins or a non-nucleotide for RNA. The difference between lengths of sequences could increase the sparsity of the TF-IDF data frame and affect the performance of our predictive model. The exploratory data analysis gave more details on the dataset (see **Table 1**). The first quartile of proteins lengths was 252 while the third quartile was 614, which means that the lengths of 50% of our combined dataset lie between 252 and 614. After all considerations, we decided to use this 50% of the dataset, containing 10,715 clean pairs, to train and test the predictive model.

2.1 Transformation of the sequence into text format

The biological sequences are sequences of successive letters without space with different lengths which are relevant to their biochemical structure and for their biological function. The bioinformaticians use the alignment process to arrange the primary structure of a protein to identify regions of similarity that may be a consequence of functional, structural, or evolutionary relationships between the sequences.

Dataset	Positive pairs	Negative pairs	#RNA	#Protein
RPI488	243	245	25	247
RPI2241	2241	2241*	841	2042
RPI12737	12,737	12737*	4636	449

**The number with star means that the negative pairs were not reported. All non-reported pairs are considered as negative.*

Table 1.
Description of different dataset used in random forest training.

This approach leaves a lot of holes in a sequence when a region from sequence of interest is not similar to the region of the other sequence. The alignment of multiple sequences is not as simple as it may seem at the first glance and the position feature of amino acids is threatened. Therefore, we propose a method which conserves the position feature of amino acids in the sequence by translating sequences into terms to apply the same representation technique for text data. T232he window with a subrange in the sequence that gives the best metrics was used and slipped through the given sequence with a fixed step, and each nucleotide (amino acid) segment was stored as a term. The shortest size of the sliding window that gave better metrics values was the size 3. As in the example below, the illustration of sequence transformation using a sliding window with size from one to four (**Figure 1**).

2.2 TF-IDF for feature engineering

The natural language processing has various types of approaches to transform the sequence of words into numerical values, such as the bag of words, words embedding, the term frequency inverse document frequency (TF-IDF), and so on. The TF-IDF measures the frequency of a term in a sequence which highly depends on the length of the sequence. The purpose of this method is to vectorize sequences [26–30]. To solve the sequence issue with the complicated alignment, TF-IDF method uses the combination of all possible terms in the dataset to have vectors of the same length with two extreme cases where TF value will be zero if the term does not appear in the dataset and 1 if all terms in the sequence are the same. The Term Frequency (TF) is used to measure how many times a term is present in a sequence and The Inverse Document Frequency assigns lower weight to frequent terms and assigns greater weight for the terms that are infrequent [31–33]. The TFIDF is the most widely used term weighting scheme. Yang and Huang [34] used it for calculating term weight according to the location and length of the

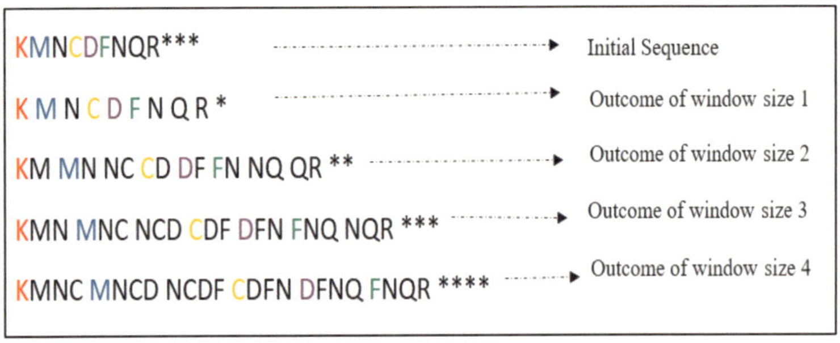

Figure 1.
Illustration of a sequence to text format using a sliding window of different sizes.

keyword and Tian Xia and Yanmei Chai [35] implemented it by calculating distribution based on local term weighting and global term weighting to improve the efficiency of IR and TC systems and many researchers used the TF-IDF for feature engineering [36–38] to solve classification problems in reasonable time, efforts, and resources.

Assuming S a set of sequences: S = {s: s is a sequence} and T a set of terms: T = {t: t is a term.

TF would be a function defined as follow:

$$TF : T * S \overset{TF}{\rightarrow} [0, 1] : (t : s) \overset{TF}{\rightarrow} TF(t, s) = \frac{Number\ of\ apprearence\ of\ t}{Number\ of\ terms\ in\ s} \tag{1}$$

Where t is a given term in a sequence s. The IDF function or normalization function which calculates the importance of a sequence in the dataset will be defined as follow:

$$IDF(S_t) : S_T \overset{IDF}{\rightarrow} \mathbb{R} : S_t \overset{IDF}{\rightarrow} IDF(S_t) = \frac{N}{S_t} \tag{2}$$

Where S_T is the set of all sequences containing the term t and N is the number of all sequences in the dataset and $s_t = |S_T|$. Thereafter, the TF-IDF is the multiplicative value of TF(t,s) and IDF(s_t)

$$TFIDF(t, s) = TF(t, s) * IDF(S_t) = \frac{N_t^s * N}{N_t * S_t} \tag{3}$$

WhereN_t^s is the number appearances of term t in a sequence s and N_t is the number of sequences containing the term t (**Figure 2**).

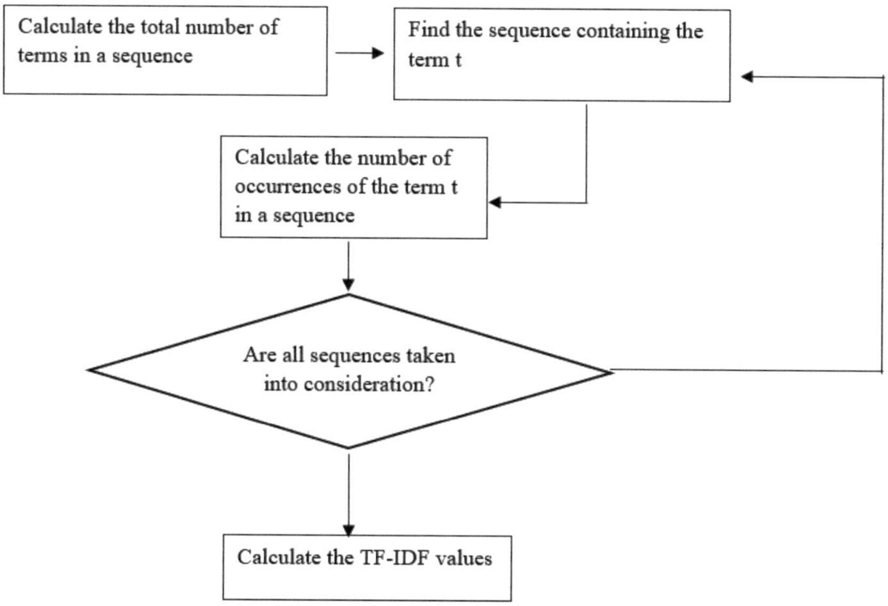

Figure 2.
The term frequency-inverse document frequency flowchart.

2.3 Feature selection

The TF-IDF method vectorises the RNA and RBP sequences and transforms them into a 2D data frame with 10,715 rows and 7461 columns. I this situation, the dimensionality reduction is required. The XgBoost method, an optimized implementation of gradient boosted decision trees in python libraries, was used to estimate the importance of TF-values. That estimation consists in comparison of all attributes to each other, to rank them based on their contribution to the general classification. Extreme gradient boosting (XGBoost) is a new method that It can take weak feature classifiers and into one strong classifier [39] due to its gradient boosting algorithm, efficiency, flexibility, and portability [40, 41]. The XGBoost was used in the literature to discover and retain the features that highly impact the prediction [42–46] and was ten time less computationally expensive compared to other popular techniques [42].

2.4 Dataset balancing

In the 10,715 samples we have, 6333 were labeled as positive samples (interacting pairs) while other 4382 were labeled as negative samples. The 1951 samples of difference between two classes are not enormous. However, most machine learning algorithms do not work very well with such imbalanced datasets [31, 47, 48]. This why we tried to train our model on unbalanced dataset and balance it thereafter. There are several techniques to balance datasets [32] but we chose to use two of them: Random Oversampling by using the bootstrapping method to increase the size of the minority class, and Under sampling that applies a nearest-neighbors algorithm [48] and "edit" the dataset by removing samples which do not agree "enough" with their neighborhood.

3. Predictive model: random Forest

The prediction of RPIs was done after training and testing the Random Forest among other classifiers. The RF is a supervised machine learning algorithm that is constructed from decision tree algorithms developed by Tin Kam Ho in 1995 [33, 34] and used to solve classification and regression problems. The random forest establishes the result according to the mean predictions of all the decision trees. A decision tree consists of decision nodes, leaf nodes, and a root node. The algorithm behind the decision tree divides the training set into branches, which further split into new branches branches until a leaf node is attained (a leaf node cannot be splitted into other branches). This sequence of branches uses the Classification And Regression Tree (CART) methodology combined to the resampling with replacement [25]. The random forest has multiple parameters that can be optimized by most of them were kept by default. Among the parameters the criterion Gini and the minimum of sample required to split fixed at two trees and hundred branches were chosen for better results.

3.1 Classification trees (Forest)

A decision tree is a way of representing knowledge obtained in the inductive learning process. The space is split using a set of conditions, and the resulting structure is the tree. Assuming we have n pairs and TF-values vectors $\{X_i\}_{i=1}^{n}$with outcomes y_i, our dataset can be presented as follow:

$$Dataset = \{(X_1,\ y_1),\ (X_2,\ y_2),\ \dots,\ (X_n,\ y_n)\} \tag{4}$$

Each TF-value vector is $X_k = (X_{k1}, X_{k2}, \dots X_{kd})$ and d is the number of TF-values from RNA and RBP altogether.

The decision tree is defined as binary process where a decision is made based on whether the TF-value X_i is inferior to a threshold t or not. This threshold depends on the node at which the decision is made. The top node contains all examples (X_n, y_n), and these examples are subdivided into children nodes according to the possibility of classification at that node. The subdivision of examples continues until every node at the bottom has examples which are in one class only.

3.2 The Gini criterion

The Random Forest as a python implementation of the scikit-learn library, this is made by the parameter 'criterion '. This parameter is the function used to measure the quality of a split and it allows users to choose between 'Gini ', or 'entropy '. We preferred the Gini criterion because computationally, entropy is more complex since it makes use of logarithms and consequently, the calculation of the Gini Index will be faster. The Gini criterion is used to measure the diversity at each tree node when the TF-value and optimal threshold are chosen. Assuming the set of all examples is S and the set of examples at the node j is Sj, then S is a partition of children node sets, i.e.:

$$S = \bigcup_1^l S_j \textit{ where l is the number of children nodes}$$

Each sample Sj is portioned into two classes C1 = interacting pair and C2 = non-interacting pair. The proportion of a sample Sj in the set of all examples and the proportion of Sj with a class Ci are respectively defined as follow:

$$P(S_j) = \frac{|S_j|}{|S|}$$
$$P(C_i|S_j) = \frac{|S_j \cap C_i|}{S} \tag{5}$$

The Gini criterion is the variation g(Sj) in the set Sj defined as follow:

$$g(S_j) = \sum_1^1 P(C_i|S_j)(1 - P(C_i|S_j)) \tag{6}$$

The variation g(Sj) reaches the maximum when the set Sj is equally divided in the class Ci and the minimum when the set Sj is just made by one of the two classes. The variation the full subdivision Sj (known as Gini Index) is defined as the weighted sum of their respective proportions in the set of all examples.

$$Gini\ Index = P(S_1)(g(S_1) + P(S_2)(g(S_2) + \dots P(S_l)(g(S_l) \tag{7}$$

3.3 The random vector

A random vector is defined as an array X of random variables defined on the same probability space. In this study the array is the TF-values vectors

$$X = (X_1, X_2 \ldots X_d) \textit{ where } X_i \textit{are column vectors} \quad (8)$$

The random y = $\{y_1, y_2, \ldots y_d\}$ with $y_i \in \{0,1\}$ is the classification of examples where 1 represent a protein-RNA interaction (RPI) while 0 represent a non-interaction. The model vector (X,y) is defined on the same probability space as the random vector X.

The goal of this predictive model is to build a classifier which predict the random vector y (classes) from random vector X (TF-values) based on the examples in the dataset from paragraph 3.1. This classifier is based on a family of classification trees and the ensemble of those trees is called Random Forest.

3.4 Ten-fold cross-validation method

The cross-validation is a resampling procedure used to evaluate machine learning models on a limited data sample. The procedure has a single parameter called k that refers to the number of groups that a given dataset is to be split into, and it is called k-fold cross-validation (k = 10 for this study). The 80% was used for the 10-fold cross validation, randomly shuffled and split into 10 groups. Among the 10 groups, only one group was kept as validation data to test the model and the remaining 9 sub-samples were used as training data. Importantly, each observation in the validation set is assigned to an individual group and stays in that group for the duration of the procedure. This means that each sample is given the opportunity to be used in the hold out set 1 time and used to train the model 9 times. The 10 results were then averaged to produce a single estimate by summarizing the mean of the model scores. The metrics we used to evaluate the model performance are Accuracy, Specificity, Sensitivity and MCC (Matthews Correlation Coefficient)

$$\text{Accuracy} = \frac{\text{TP} + \text{TN}}{\text{TP} + \text{TN} + \text{FN} + \text{TN}}$$

$$\text{Specificity} = \frac{\text{TN}}{\text{TN} + \text{FP}}$$

$$\text{Sensitivity} = \frac{\text{TP}}{\text{TP} + \text{FN}}$$

$$\text{MCC} = \frac{\text{TP} * \text{TN} - \text{FP} * \text{FN}}{\sqrt{(\text{TP} + \text{TN})(\text{FP} + \text{FN})(\text{TP} + \text{FN})(\text{TP} + \text{FP})}} \quad (9)$$

Where TP, FP, TN, and FN stand for True Positive, False Positive, True Negative and False Negative respectively.

3.5 Independent test

The remaining 20% of the dataset was used to test the classifier performance to the unseen data. This test dataset was completely independent of the data sample used in 10-fold cross validation. The goal was to train the Random Forest with parameters having the best performance on new data.

4. Results and discussion

We have applied the sliding window approach to transform RNA and protein sequences into text format using different window's sizes starting from size 2. We constated that there was not much difference between the model performance when using a sliding window size of 3,4 or 5 and the performance started decreasing at window size of 6. Therefore, we chose the window's size 3 because it gives the best results in less time. After we applied the TF-IDF to the dataset we got a data frame of 10,715 rows and 7461 attributes. The Random Forest applied to this dataset gave a good performance with a scope of improvement because all 7461 features do not have the same importance in the prediction. We applied the XgBoost algorithm to select the best features. The best threshold showed that 232 features contribute to the prediction at 0.2% at least. The performances of different classifiers are summarized in **Table 2**.

The receiver operating characteristic (ROC) curves of the three classifiers confirms our preference of the Random Forest to other classifiers. The Area under the curve is 0.98, 0.95 and 0.93 for Random Forest, Logistic Regression and Multinomial Naïve Bayesian respectively (**Figure 3**). Sometimes, one algorithm can overperform other algorithms for one metric measure and loses for other metrics. But in this study, the

Classifiers	10-Fold cross validation				Independent test			
	Spe	*Sen*	*Acc*	*MCC*	*Spec*	*Sen*	*Acc*	*MCC*
RF	0.96	0.94	0.95	0.92	0.95	0.94	0.94	0.90
LR	0.96	0.89	0.92	0.84	0.93	0.89	0.91	0.83
MNB	0.95	0.89	0.92	0.84	0.93	0.88	0.91	0.82

RF = Random Forest; LR = Logistic Regression; MNB = Multinomial Naïve Bayesian.

Table 2.
Comparative summary of three different predictive models.

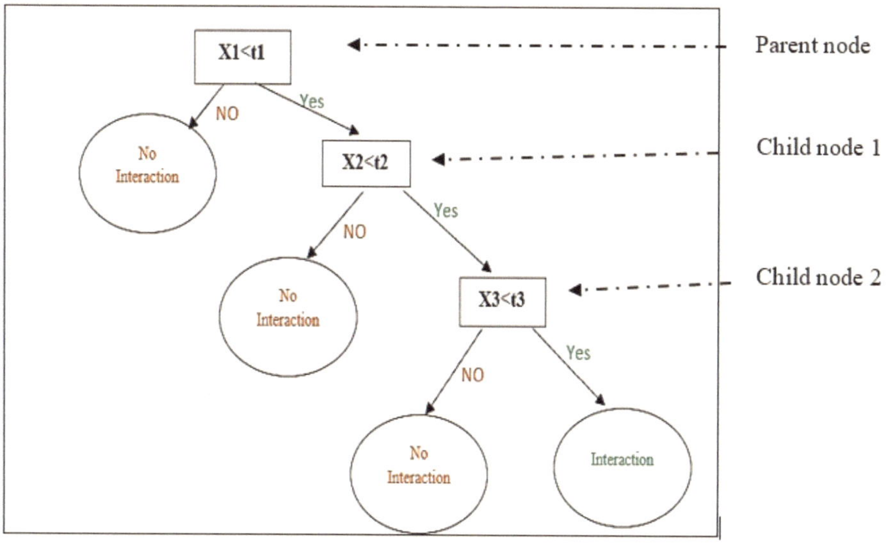

Figure 3.
Illustration of classification trees with three nodes. The thresholds ti depends on each note and are learned during the training process.

Random Forest overperformed other two classifiers in all metrics and more importantly for Matthew Correlation Coefficient (MCC) because it is an ensemble-based algorithm using the resampling with replacement method to reduce variance. This method makes that the Random Forest takes a lot of time to be trained but it is worth it because: a tree-based learning algorithm, on large datasets, allows to quantitative and qualitative input variables, can be immune to redundant variables or variables with high correlation which may lead to overfitting in other learning algorithms and has few parameters to tune (**Figures 4** and 5).

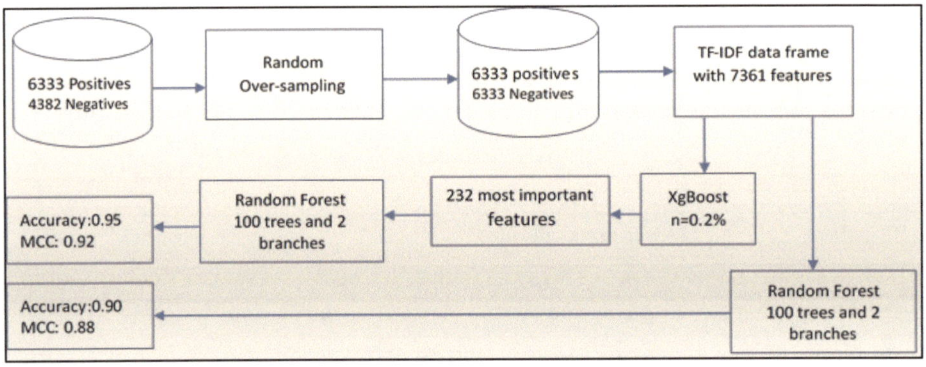

Figure 4.
A systematics review of imbalanced data challenges and dimensionality reduction.

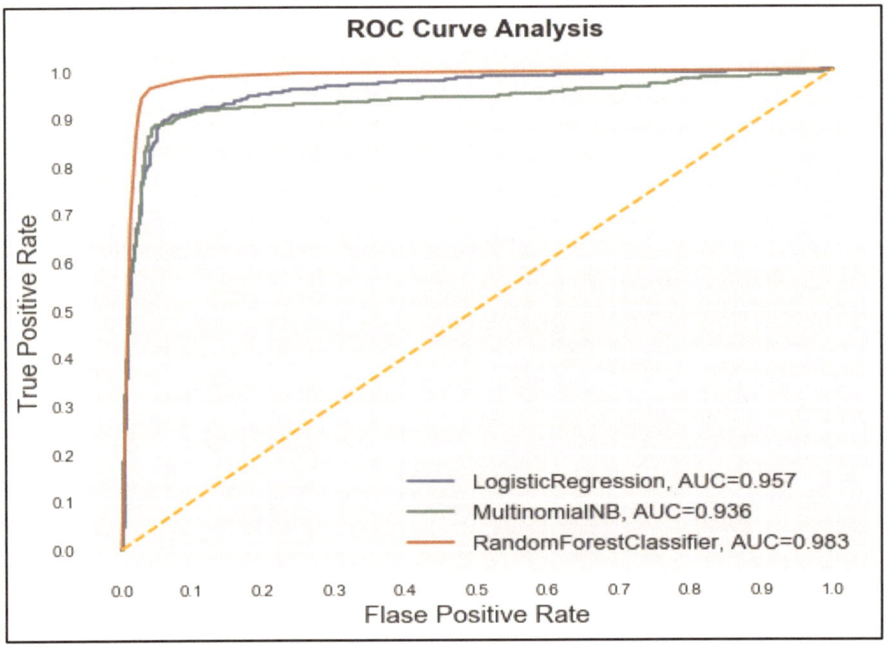

Figure 5.
Representation of ROC of the AUC for three classifiers showing that the random Forest curve is higher than other classifiers.

5. Conclusions

The Term Frequency Inverse Document Frequency borrowed from natural language processing was combined with the sliding window to transform the RNA and protein sequences into a data frame of numerical values and 232 most contributing TF-values were selected using the XgBoost feature importance. Based on these features, we trained the Random Forest classier on 10,132 samples and tested it on 2534 remaining samples. The results in the **Table 2** show that the Random Forest overperformed all other predictive models that we trained on this dataset for comparison such as Logistic Regression and Multinomial Naïve Bayesian. The highest AUC for the Random Forest, combined with the high specificity and sensitivity, provides an indication of its ability to correctly predict all classes in large datasets. The Random Forest is computationally expensive, but there is a significant performance difference compared to other classifiers which is worth the training time.

Acknowledgements

This study was supported by Visualization and Computation Advancing Research (ViCAR) Center and funded by National Science Fund (NSF).

Author details

Eugene Uwiragiye and Kristen L. Rhinehardt*
Computational Data Science and Engineering, North Carolina Agricultural and Technical State University, Greensboro, NC, United States of America

*Address all correspondence to: klrhineh@ncat.edu

References

[1] Jain DS, Gupte SR, Aduri R. A data driven model for predicting rna-protein interactions based on gradient boosting machine. Scientific Reports. 2018;**8**(1):1-10

[2] Licatalosi DD, Darnell RB. RNA processing and its regulation: Global insights into biological networks. Nature Reviews Genetics. 2010;**11**(1):75-87

[3] Kishore S, Luber S, Zavolan M. Deciphering the role of RNA-binding proteins in the post-transcriptional control of gene expression. Briefings in Functional Genomics. 2010;**9**(5–6):391-404

[4] Beckmann BM et al. The RNA-binding proteomes from yeast to man harbour conserved enigmRBPs. Nature Communications. 2015;**6**(1):1-9

[5] Allers J, Shamoo Y. Structure-based analysis of protein-RNA interactions using the program ENTANGLE. Journal of Molecular Biology. 2001;**311**(1):75-86

[6] Terribilini M et al. Prediction of RNA binding sites in proteins from amino acid sequence. RNA. 2006;**12**(8): 1450-1462

[7] Kim OT, Yura K, Go N. Amino acid residue doublet propensity in the protein–RNA interface and its application to RNA interface prediction. Nucleic Acids Research. 2006;**34**(22): 6450-6460

[8] Wang H, Wu P. Prediction of RNA-protein interactions using conjoint triad feature and chaos game representation. Bioengineered. 2018;**9**(1):242-251

[9] Mercer TR, Mattick JS. Structure and function of long noncoding RNAs in epigenetic regulation. Nature Structural & Molecular Biology. 2013;**20**(3): 300-307

[10] Pancaldi V, Bähler J. In silico characterization and prediction of global protein–mRNA interactions in yeast. Nucleic Acids Research. 2011;**39**(14): 5826-5836

[11] Bellucci M et al. Predicting protein associations with long noncoding RNAs. Nature Methods. 2011;**8**(6):444-445

[12] Muppirala UK, Honavar VG, Dobbs D. Predicting RNA-protein interactions using only sequence information. BMC Bioinformatics. 2011;**12**(1):1-11

[13] Lewis BA et al. PRIDB: A protein–RNA interface database. Nucleic Acids Research. 2010;**39**(suppl_1):D277-D282

[14] Agostini F et al. Cat RAPID omics: A web server for large-scale prediction of protein–RNA interactions. Bioinformatics. 2013;**29**(22):2928-2930

[15] Agostini F et al. X-inactivation: Quantitative predictions of protein interactions in the Xist network. Nucleic Acids Research. 2013;**41**(1):e31-e31

[16] Zhan Z-H et al. BGFE: A deep learning model for ncRNA-protein interaction predictions based on improved sequence information. International Journal of Molecular Sciences. 2019;**20**(4):978

[17] Suresh V et al. RPI-Pred: Predicting ncRNA-protein interaction using sequence and structural information. Nucleic Acids Research. 2015;**43**(3): 1370-1379

[18] Liu H et al. LPI-NRLMF: lncRNA-protein interaction prediction by neighborhood regularized logistic matrix factorization. Oncotarget. 2017;**8**(61): 103975

[19] Cheng S et al. DM-RPIs: Predicting ncRNA-protein interactions using stacked ensembling strategy. Computational Biology and Chemistry. 2019;**83**:107088

[20] Zhao Q et al. IRWNRLPI: Integrating random walk and neighborhood regularized logistic matrix factorization for lncRNA-protein interaction prediction. Frontiers in Genetics. 2018;**9**:239

[21] Chen X et al. BNPMDA: Bipartite network projection for MiRNA–disease association prediction. Bioinformatics. 2018;**34**(18):3178-3186

[22] Hu H et al. HLPI-ensemble: Prediction of human lncRNA-protein interactions based on ensemble strategy. RNA Biology. 2018;**15**(6):797-806

[23] Pan X et al. IPMiner: hidden ncRNA-protein interaction sequential pattern mining with stacked autoencoder for accurate computational prediction. BMC Genomics. 2016;**17**(1):1-14

[24] Zhan Z-H et al. Accurate prediction of ncRNA-protein interactions from the integration of sequence and evolutionary information. Frontiers in Genetics. 2018; **9**:458

[25] Yuan J et al. NPInter v2. 0: An updated database of ncRNA interactions. Nucleic Acids Research. 2014;**42**(D1): D104-D108

[26] Trstenjak B, Mikac S, Donko D. KNN with TF-IDF based framework for text categorization. Procedia Engineering. 2014;**69**:1356-1364

[27] Joachims T. Text categorization with support vector machines: Learning with many relevant features. In: European Conference on Machine Learning. Berlin, Heidelberg: Springer; 1998

[28] Yang Y, Liu X. A re-examination of text categorization methods. In: Proceedings of the 22nd Annual International ACM SIGIR Conference on Research and Development in Information Retrieval. 1999

[29] Soucy P, Mineau GW. Beyond TFIDF weighting for text categorization in the vector space model. In: International Joint Conferences on Artificial Intelligence Organization. Vol. 5. 2005

[30] Xu G et al. Improved TFIDF weighting for imbalanced biomedical text classification. Energy Procedia. 2011;**11**:2360-2367

[31] Beckmann M, Ebecken NF, de Lima BSP. A KNN undersampling approach for data balancing. Journal of Intelligent Learning Systems and Applications. 2015;7(04):104

[32] Santos MS et al. A new cluster-based oversampling method for improving survival prediction of hepatocellular carcinoma patients. Journal of Biomedical Informatics. 2015;**58**:49-59

[33] Li B-Q et al. Prediction of protein-protein interaction sites by random forest algorithm with mRMR and IFS. PLoS One. 2012;7(8):e43927

[34] Zhu C, Cheng G, Wang K. Big data analytics for program popularity prediction in broadcast TV industries. IEEE Access. 2017;5:24593-24601

[35] Tian, X., and W. Tong. An improvement to tf: Term distribution-based term weight algorithm. 2010 Second International Conference on Networks Security, Wireless Communications and Trusted Computing. 2010. IEEE

[36] Liu L, Peng T. Clustering-based method for positive and unlabeled text

categorization enhanced by improved TFIDF. Journal Information Science Engineering. 2014;**30**(5):1463-1481

[37] Qu S, Wang S, Zou Y. Improvement of text feature selection method based on tfidf. In: 2008 International Seminar on Future Information Technology and Management Engineering. IEEE; 2008

[38] Goswami P, Kamath V. The DF-ICF algorithm-modified TF-IDF. International Journal of Computer Applications. 2014;**93**(13)

[39] Li D et al. Feature selection and model fusion approach for predicting urban macro travel time. Mathematical Problems in Engineering. 2020;**2020**

[40] Brownlee J. XGBoost With python: Gradient boosted trees with XGBoost and scikit-learn. Machine Learning Mastery; 2016

[41] Chang W et al. A machine-learning-based prediction method for hypertension outcomes based on medical data. Diagnostics. 2019;**9**(4):178

[42] Chen T, Guestrin C. Xgboost: A scalable tree boosting system. In: Proceedings of the 22nd Acm Sigkdd International Conference on Knowledge Discovery and Data Mining. 2016

[43] He X et al. Practical lessons from predicting clicks on ads at facebook. In: Proceedings of the Eighth International Workshop on Data Mining for Online Advertising. 2014

[44] Pal A, Shrivastava N, Tripathi P. Comparison of Classification Algorithms Using Machine Learning. 2019

[45] Horrell M. Wide Boosting. arXiv preprint arXiv:2007.09855, 2020

[46] Bennett J, Lanning S. The netflix prize. In: Proceedings of KDD Cup and Workshop. New York; 2007

[47] Domingues I et al. Evaluation of oversampling data balancing techniques in the context of ordinal classification. In: 2018 International Joint Conference on Neural Networks (IJCNN). IEEE; 2018

[48] Rodríguez JP, Corrales DC, Corrales JC. A process for increasing the samples of coffee rust through machine learning methods. International Journal of Agricultural and Environmental Information Systems (IJAEIS). 2018;**9**(2):32-52